Syncope and Transient Loss of Consciousness

MULTIDISCIPLINARY MANAGEMENT

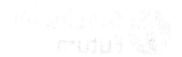

Syncope and Transient Loss of Consciousness

MULTIDISCIPLINARY
MANAGEMENT

Edited by

David G Benditt, MD, FACC, FRCP(C), FHRS
Cardiac Arrhythmia Center, Department of Medicine, Cardiovascular Division,
University of Minnesota, Minneapolis, USA

Michele Brignole, MD, FESC
Head, Department of Cardiology and Arrhythmologic Center, Ospedali Riuniti,
Lavagna, Italy

Antonio Raviele, MD, FESC
Head, Cardiovascular Department, Umberto I Hospital, Venice-Mestre, Italy

Wouter Wieling, MD, PhD
Department of Medicine, Academic Medical Centre, University of Amsterdam,
Amsterdam, The Netherlands

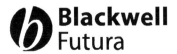

© 2007 Blackwell Publishing
Blackwell Futura is an imprint of Blackwell Publishing

Blackwell Publishing, Inc., 350 Main Street, Malden, Massachusetts 02148-5020, USA
Blackwell Publishing Ltd, 9600 Garsington Road, Oxford OX4 2DQ, UK
Blackwell Science Asia Pty Ltd, 550 Swanston Street, Carlton, Victoria 3053, Australia

First published 2007

1   2007

ISBN: 978-1-4051-7625-5

Library of Congress Cataloging-in-Publication Data

Syncope and transient loss of consciousness : multidisciplinary management / edited by David
G. Benditt . . . [et al.].
    p. ; cm.
    Includes bibliographical references and index.
    ISBN 978-1-4051-7625-5 (alk. paper)
1. Syncope (Pathology)   2. Loss of consciousness.   I. Benditt, David G.

[DNLM: 1. Syncope–diagnosis.   2. Syncope–etiology.   3. Syncope–therapy.
WB 182 S9913 2007]

RB150.L67S82 2007
155.9′3–dc22
                                            2007021631

A catalogue record for this title is available from the British Library

Commissioning Editor: Gina Almond
Development Editor: Fiona Pattison
Production Controller: Debbie Wyer

Set in 9.5/12pt Palatino by Aptara Inc., New Delhi, India
Printed and bound in Spain by Graphycems, Navarra

For further information on Blackwell Publishing, visit our website:
www.blackwellcardiology.com

The publisher's policy is to use permanent paper from mills that operate a sustainable forestry
policy, and which has been manufactured from pulp processed using acid-free and elementary
chlorine-free practices. Furthermore, the publisher ensures that the text paper and cover board
used have met acceptable environmental accreditation standards.

Contents

Part 3 Specific conditions

Part 4 Economic and research aspects

Part 5 Current controversies and future directions

Contributors

Paolo Alboni, MD, FESC
Chief
Division of Cardiology and Arrhythmologic
    Center
Cento
Italy

Dietrich Andresen, Prof Dr Med
Medical Director
Head of the Department of Cardiology
Berlin
Germany

David G Benditt, MD, FACC,
FRCP(C), FHRS
Cardiac Arrhythmia Center
Department of Medicine
Cardiovascular Division
University of Minnesota
Minneapolis
USA

Jean-Jacques Blanc, MD
Department of Cardiology
Hôpital De La Cavale Blanche
Brest University Hospital
Brest
France

Michele Brignole, MD, FESC
Head
Department of Cardiology and
    Arrhythmologic Center
Ospedali Riuniti
Lavagna
Italy

Hugh Calkins, MD, FACC, FAHA
Professor of Medicine
Professor of Pediatrics
Director of the Arrhythmia Service; and
Clinical Electrophysiology Laboratory, Director of
    the ARVD Program Johns Hopkins Hospital
Baltimore
USA

A John Camm, MD FRCP, FACC, FESC
St. George's University of London
London
UK

Maurizio Dinelli, MD
Division of Cardiology and
    Arrhythmologic Center
Cento
Italy

Hugo Ector, MD, PhD, FESC
Departments of Cardiology and
    Cardiovascular Rehabilitation
Gasthuisberg University Hospital
University of Leuven (KU Leuven)
Leuven
Belgium

Adam Fitzpatrick, MD, FRCP, FACC
Manchester Heart Centre
Manchester Royal Infirmary
Manchester
UK

Franco Giada, MD
Electrophysiologist
Cardiologist
Cardiovascular Department
Umberto I Hospital
Venice/Mestre
Italy

Blair P Grubb, MD
Professor of Medicine and Pediatrics
Division of Cardiovascular Medicine
Department of Medicine
University of Toledo
Toledo
Ohio
USA

Juan C Guzman, MD
Fellow in Syncope and Autonomic Disorders
MSc Candidate in Health Research
    Methodology
Department of Medicine
Faculty of Health Sciences
McMaster University/Hamilton
    Health Sciences
Hamilton
Ontario
Canada

Rose Anne Kenny, MD, FESC
Head of Department of Medical Gerontology
Trinity College
Dublin
Ireland

Andrew D Krahn, MD, FRCP(C)
Program Director, Electrophysiology
  Training Program
Professor, Division of Cardiology
University of Western Ontario, London, Ontario,
Canada

Chu-Pak Lau, MD, FRCP, FACC
William MW Mong Professor in Cardiology
Cardiology Division, Department of Medicine
Queen Mary Hospital
University of Hong Kong
Hong Kong Special Administrative Region
China

Kathy L Lee, MBBS, FRCP, FACC
Cardiology Division
Department of Medicine
Queen Mary Hospital
University of Hong Kong
Hong Kong Special Administrative Region
China

Christopher Mathias, DPhil, DSc,
FRCP, FMedSci
Autonomic Unit
National Hospital for Neurology and
  Neurosurgery
Queen Sqaure; and
Institute of Neurology
University College London
London
UK

Suneet Mittal, MD
Division of Cardiology and the
  Arrhythmia Institute
The St. Luke's-Roosevelt Hospital Center
Columbia University College of Physicians &
  Surgeons
New York
USA

Carlos Morillo, MD FRCPC, FACC, FHRS,
FESC
Professor Department of Medicine
Director Arrhythmia Service, Cardiology
  Division
Department of Medicine, Faculty of Health
  Sciences
McMaster University/Hamilton Health Sciences
Hamilton
Ontario
Canada

Angel Moya, MD, PhD
Chief of Arrhythmia Unit
Cardiology Department
Hospital Universitari Vall d'Hebrón
Barcelona
Spain

Christina M Murray, MD
Fellow, Cardiovascular Section
University of Oklahoma Health Sciences Center
Oklahoma City
Oklahoma
USA

Gerald V Naccarelli, MD, FACC
Penn State Heart and Vascular Institute
Penn State University College of Medicine
Hershey
Pennsylvania
USA

Brian Olshansky, MD, FACC
Professor of Medicine
University of Iowa Hospitals
Iowa City
USA

Antonio Raviele, MD, FESC
Cardiovascular Department
Umberto I Hospital
Venice-Mestre
Italy

Tony Reybrouck, PhD
Departments of Cardiology and Cardiovascular
  Rehabilitation
Gasthuisberg University Hospital
University of Leuven (KU Leuven)
Leuven
Belgium

Dwight W Reynolds, MD, FACC, FHRS
University of Oklahoma
Health Sciences Center
Professor and Chief, Cardiovascular Section
Oklahoma City
Oklahoma
USA

François P Sarasin, MD, MSc
Emergency Division
Department of Internal Medicine
Hôpital Cantonal
University of Geneva Medical School
Geneva
Switzerland

Anna Serletis, MD
The Libin Cardiovascular Institute of Alberta
University of Calgary
Calgary
Alberta
Canada

Robert S Sheldon, MD, PhD, FRCP(C)
The Libin Cardiovascular Institute of Alberta
University of Calgary
Calgary
Alberta
Canada

Win K Shen, MD
Division of Cardiovascular Diseases
Department of Internal Medicine
Mayo Clinic College of Medicine
Rochester
Minnesota
USA

Richard Sutton, DScMed, FRCP, FACC,
FESC, FANA, FHRS
Consultant Cardiologist
Royal Brompton and Chelsea and Westminster
  Hospitals
London
UK

Roland D Thijs, MD
Department of Neurology and Clinical
  Neurophysiology
Leiden University Medical Centre
Leiden
The Netherlands

Hung-Fat Tse, MD, FRCP, FACC
Cardiology Division
Department of Medicine
Queen Mary Hospital
University of Hong Kong
Hong Kong Special Administrative Region
China

Gert van Dijk, MD, PhD
Department of Neurology and Clinical
  Neurophysiology
Leiden University Medical Centre
Leiden
The Netherlands

W Wieling, MD, PhD
Department of Medicine
Academic Medical Centre
University of Amsterdam
Meibergdreef
Amsterdam
The Netherlands

Preface

Optimizing management of syncope remains a challenge. The fundamental problem is that "syncope" is only one of the many causes of transient loss of consciousness (TLOC). Other causes of TLOC, including epilepsy, intoxications, and concussions, are also important medical conditions but are distinct from syncope. Consequently, when confronted with a patient who presents with an apparent self-terminating "collapse" or "blackout," the essential first step is ascertaining whether the problem was indeed syncope (i.e., a period of self-limited cerebral hypoperfusion); only then can one reasonably begin to contemplate which of the many potential causes of syncope was at fault.

Syncope is a fleeting symptom only rarely witnessed by a medically experienced bystander, and in almost every case the patient has fully recovered when finally seen. As a result, important components of the event history may not be reported clearly, if at all. Furthermore, the subsequent evaluation must rely on identifying comorbidities (if any) and discerning susceptibilities that could have been responsible for loss of consciousness. In such a setting, the diagnosis is one of inference; the relationship between a detected abnormality and spontaneous symptoms is largely presumptive, with varying degrees of uncertainty remaining.

Further complicating the clinical dilemma is the fact that patients with TLOC/syncope lack a single avenue for seeking diagnosis and treatment. Since a "collapse" may occur in any age group (from early childhood to the elderly) and in a variety of settings (at home, at work, at school, or during recreation or athletic activity), and may be associated with none or any number of underlying comorbidities, the initial referral for assessment may be directed to any of several different medical specialties. Thus, as things currently stand in most places, there is no single structure for syncope care. General practitioners, emergency physicians, cardiologists, neurologists, pediatricians, or geriatricians may be confronted with the initial evaluation, and their experience in dealing with TLOC/syncope may vary considerably.

Given recognition that TLOC/syncope is a frequently encountered problem (about 1% of emergency department visits) and may contribute importantly to diminishing quality of life, increasing propensity to physical injury, or even to increasing mortality risk, considerable attention has been directed toward improving its management. In large measure, the European Society of Cardiology (ESC) Syncope Guideline initiative led the way. Subsequently, studies from various parts of the world, many being multicenter randomized and/or controlled trials, have contributed to our better understanding of a wide range of pertinent issues, including:

- criteria for diagnosis of the cause of syncope from history and physical examination;
- optimal diagnostic testing strategies;
- new insights into treatment options; and
- the need for a multidisciplinary structured approach to TLOC/syncope management, including development of a multidisciplinary practice guideline.

This volume was designed with a solitary goal in mind: to provide for the broad spectrum of individuals and expertise currently responsible for caring for TLOC/syncope patients—a succinct, timely, and practical update on diagnostic and treatment strategies. To this end, incorporated within each focused chapter are the latest concepts and most current citations. Every effort has been made to provide easily readable practical recommendations (evidence-based when possible) that amplify and extend those provided in the ESC guideline document. Our hope is that the reader will find this to be a user-friendly volume replete with the latest meaningful clinical tips. Finally, we hope that this effort will be viewed as forming part of a necessarily evolving foundation upon which a true multinational, multidisciplinary TLOC/syncope practice guideline may ultimately be constructed.

David G Benditt, MD
Michele Brignole, MD
Antonio Raviele, MD
Wouter Wieling, MD
May 1, 2007

PART 1

Syncope and TLOC overview

CHAPTER 1

Definition and classification of syncope and transient loss of consciousness

Jean-Jacques Blanc

Syncope is a common complaint responsible for up to 1% of admissions in emergency departments in Europe [1–4]. During the last two decades cardiologists have become the specialists most involved in developing the diagnosis and treatment strategies for patients with presumed syncope, but they are not alone; many other physicians of various specialities are interested in the management of patients with syncope, including neurology, internal medicine, and geriatrics among others.

In order to establish a uniform standard of care for syncope patients despite the participation of diverse specialities, it is essential that there be a common language. Perhaps most critical in this regard is a clear understanding of what "syncope" is, and why other conditions that cause real or apparent transient loss of consciousness (TLOC) are not classified as "syncope." Unfortunately, a widely acceptable uniform definition does not currently exist.

The aim of this chapter is to develop a definition of syncope that can be defended and that might prove to be acceptable for use across multiple medical specialties. To this end, the subject is approached through a series of questions and responses.

Is syncope a symptom?

The word "symptom" is generally accepted to mean "a sensation or change in health function experienced by a patient." This definition certainly applies to "syncope," but this, of course, is insufficient to fully characterize the term "syncope."

Syncope is a symptom, but is it the same as TLOC?

The notion of TLOC is certainly included in the etymology of the word "syncope" that is derived from an ancient Greek word, meaning "interrupt."

Syncope and Transient Loss of Consciousness, 1st edition. Edited by David G Benditt *et al.*
© 2007 Blackwell Publishing, ISBN: 978-1-4051-7625-5.

Therefore, it is reasonable to assume that TLOC must be an essential element of "true" syncope.

Determining whether TLOC actually occurred in a given clinical situation may not be easy; it can only be derived from careful evaluation of the history taken from the patient or from eyewitnesses. In the absence of TLOC the diagnosis of syncope should be excluded. However, the concept of TLOC is much broader than just "syncope." TLOC incorporates many other conditions that cause self-limited loss of consciousness but are not due to cerebral hypoperfusion (e.g., epilepsy, concussion, and intoxication). For example, a boxer who is "knocked out" can be considered to have experienced TLOC but cannot be considered as having had syncope. A patient with a toxic coma has TLOC but again cannot be considered as having had syncope. Some patients with psychogenic disorders mimic TLOC but they cannot be considered to have syncope.

Thus, we can at this stage conclude that syncope is a form of TLOC, but the two are not entirely the same. Something more should be added to this definition to fit with what is considered syncope by clinicians.

Syncope is a symptom encompassing a TLOC, but is it spontaneous?

Addition of the word "spontaneous" is necessary to exclude from the field of syncope patients with concussion (e.g., head trauma) or intoxication who require a completely different therapeutic strategy. However, in some cases, "real" syncope can lead to severe head trauma and sometimes it is difficult to determine the real primary cause. Observations by eyewitnesses may be helpful and should be sought.

Syncope is a symptom defined as a transient spontaneous loss of consciousness, but is the onset rapid?

The notion of rapid onset is ambiguous but perhaps it can be agreed that in the case of syncope the time between the onset of premonitory symptoms and the loss of consciousness is relatively brief (i.e., no more than a few dozens of seconds). Intoxications would be expected to take longer, whereas epileptic fits would be indistinguishable, in terms of abruptness of TLOC, from true syncope. Thus, the notion of rapid onset is per se insufficient to exclude some of the causes of TLOC and something more should be added to the syncope definition in order to be more precise.

Syncope is a symptom defined as a transient spontaneous loss of consciousness with a rapid onset, but is it self-limited and complete with usually a prompt recovery?

This addition is crucial. It includes two major concepts. The first is the notion of a "self-limited symptom," which means that patients recover their consciousness without any external medical interventions, such as prolonged resuscitation maneuvers including electrical cardioversion. In this latter instance, patients should be classified as having had an aborted sudden death, which is not syncope. A second example is of coma, particularly hypoglycemia, which needs a medical intervention to reverse. Thus, the "self-limited" concept excludes some conditions that result in TLOC but are not syncope.

The second concept stated here is the notion of "complete and usually prompt recovery." This element of the puzzle does not on its own totally discriminate between syncope and some types of TLOC, but it can help. For example, patients with epileptic seizures or coma usually recover slowly and in the case of certain seizures they may remain disoriented for a lengthy period of time.

The "complete and usually prompt recovery" addition tends to restrict the differential diagnosis to what "syncope" is generally considered to be in the broad medical community. But is it really enough? This definition excludes coma, concussion, resuscitated sudden death, "pseudo" TLOC, etc., but not epilepsy, which is not considered to be syncope by most medical practitioners. Something should be added to the definition to exclude this limitation.

Syncope is a symptom defined as a transient spontaneous loss of consciousness with a rapid onset, and a self-limited, complete, and usually prompt recovery in which the underlying mechanism is a transient global cerebral hypoperfusion

This is certainly the most difficult and controversial part of the definition. How could "global cerebral hypoperfusion" be documented in patients with syncope outside of a specially designed laboratory (which is not of course the usual situation)? It is obvious that we do not yet have at our disposal an ambulatory monitor capable of recording cerebral perfusion changes in free-living individuals; consequently, cerebral hypoperfusion can only be suspected based on indirect factors. On the other hand, at this stage of the evolving definition, there remain only two contenders that are consistent with the above-mentioned definition prior to adding the concept that "the underlying mechanism is a transient global cerebral hypoperfusion"; these two are "syncope" or "seizure."

In the case of epileptic seizure, there is a self-terminated TLOC but the underlying mechanism is abnormal diffuse brain electrical hyperactivity. However, since we do not have a readily deployed long-term ambulatory electroencephalographic monitor, our ability to definitively distinguish between seizure and syncope is limited. Fortunately, in most cases, the clinical picture permits differentiating between syncope (the only TLOC due to global cerebral hypoperfusion) and seizure; in fact, confusion between the two entities is (arguably) relatively rare in everyday practice. The main clinical arguments for each of the two entities are summarized in the guidelines on syncope of the European Society of Cardiology [5].

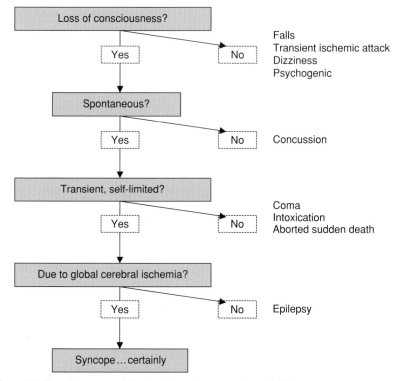

Figure 1.1 Flowchart summarizing the diagnosis strategy from TLOC to syncope.

Syncope is a symptom defined as a transient spontaneous loss of consciousness with a rapid onset, and self-limited, complete, and usually prompt recovery the underlying mechanism of which is a transient global cerebral hypoperfusion. Is this definition adequate?

This definition seems to correspond to the generally accepted view of syncope by the medical community, not just cardiologists. For example, neurologists in their vast majority do not consider that epilepsy is syncope [6].

This last iteration of the definition is very close to the one adopted by the Task Force of the European Society of Cardiology in charge of the guidelines on syncope [5]. The only concept that is not included in the current definition but present in the European Society of Cardiology's definition is "the loss of postural tone." In reality, this latter point is not very helpful, as all patients with TLOC (not exclusively those with syncope) have a "loss of postural tone."

It is evident that new data on pathophysiology of TLOC or new physiologic monitoring devices can modify the proposed definition of syncope, but it seems unlikely that it will be markedly changed. Unfortunately, however, there is a long way to go before there is acceptance of the importance of a careful definition. For example, in the recently published American College of

Cardiology/American Heart Association scientific statement [7], the definition of syncope is just limited to saying, "syncope is a symptom defined as a transient loss of consciousness." Therefore, in the eyes of the official bodies of US cardiology, TLOC and syncope are equivalent. This apparent failure to differentiate between TLOC and syncope clearly promotes long-standing confusion and leads to imprecise thinking with regard to patient management.

Conclusion

To develop an optimum uniform management strategy for any condition, a minimum requirement is clear understanding of what the condition encompasses. In the case of syncope, this level of understanding remains to be achieved. In this chapter the basic elements that characterize the syndrome of syncope have been examined. Based on consideration of these elements, a clinically applicable definition has been proposed. From this assessment it should be evident that syncope is only one of the many causes of TLOC (Figure 1.1) and that, before a final determination of the cause of a patient's symptoms can be offered, it is crucial to first ascertain whether syncope had indeed occurred or whether the apparent loss of consciousness was one of the many other conditions lying within the larger TLOC umbrella.

References

1 Blanc JJ, L'Her C, Touiza A, *et al*. Prospective evaluation and outcome of patients admitted for syncope over a 1 year period. *Eur Heart J* 2002;**23**:815–20.
2 Ammirati F, Colivicchi F, Minardi G, *et al*. Gestione della sincope in ospedale: studio OESIL. *G Ital Cardiol* 1999;**29**:533–9.
3 Farwell D, Sulke N. How do we diagnose syncope? *J Cardiovasc Electrophysiol* 2002;**13**:9–13.
4 Disertori M, Brignole M, Menozzi C, *et al*. Management of patients with syncope referred urgently to general hospitals. *Europace* 2003;**5**:283–91.
5 Brignole M, Alboni P, Benditt DG, *et al*. Guidelines on management (diagnosis and treatment) of syncope. *Eur Heart J* 2001;**22**:1256–306.
6 Thijs RD, Wieling W, Kaufmann H, van Dijk G. Defining and classifying syncope. *Clin Auton Res* 2004;**14**(suppl 1):4–8.
7 Strickberger SA, Benson DW, Jr, Biaggioni I, *et al*. AHA/ACC scientific statement on the evaluation of syncope. *J Am Coll Cardiol* 2006;**47**:473–84.

CHAPTER 2

Epidemiologic aspects of transient loss of consciousness/syncope

Robert S Sheldon, Anna Serletis

Introduction

Syndromes of transient loss of consciousness (TLOC) pose considerable challenges to health care systems. This is because of their range of etiologies, high lifetime incidence, and frequent mismatch between their prevalence, lethality, and ease of treatment. Simply put, benign causes are common, and potentially treatable and lethal causes are infrequent.

A quantitative appreciation of the epidemiology of TLOC is needed in order to permit design of clinical trials, diagnostic strategies, and health services delivery. Given the sporadically recurring nature of these syndromes, we also need a sense of their natural history and their comparative epidemiologies in the community and the clinic. This is because, although sensitivity and specificity usually define diagnostic tests, they are only marginally helpful in knowing how to use tests optimally. The truly useful measures are the predictive values, and these depend on the prevalence of the competing diagnoses.

This review is by necessity brief. A comprehensive, highly accessible, and contemporary review of the field appeared recently [1].

Review of epidemiologic principles

The usual epidemiologic terms of prevalence (the proportion of people with the disease) and incidence (the proportion of people acquiring the disease in a sampling interval) are difficult to use in characterizing TLOC syndromes. Strictly speaking, the prevalence of TLOC is close to zero because people spend so little time unconscious during a TLOC or faint. Furthermore, syncope syndromes start presenting at characteristic times of life, and first faints in these syndromes continue to occur over the years [2–5]. The terms such as cumulative proportion, cumulative event rate, or cumulative incidence are more appropriate. Finally, what we measure depends in large part on where we measure it.

Syncope and Transient Loss of Consciousness, 1st edition. Edited by David G Benditt *et al.*
© 2007 Blackwell Publishing, ISBN: 978-1-4051-7625-5.

Community prevalence of syncope

Most studies have ignored the age dependence of syncope, relying on either longitudinal surveys in specific demographic groups or cumulative recalled syncope spells in longitudinal surveys. Several studies [1, review] in the mid-twentieth century comprising generally young people reported that the recollected lifetime cumulative incidence was 18–34%; that is, up to a third of young people admitted to having had at least one syncope spell. Dermksian and Lamb [6] gave a self-reporting questionnaire to 3000 US Air Force personnel, and only 7% admitted to having fainted. Given the danger of losing consciousness during flying, this apparent difficulty with recall is not surprising.

The first Framingham study [7] followed 5029 adults, aged 30–62 years, for 26 years. Only 3.2% admitted to even one syncope spell during that time, and of these only 4% recalled having fainted as a child. These results are in stark contrast to both earlier and later studies, and they suggest that either the Framingham population is highly atypical or the syncope was either not recalled or deeply discounted by aging adults during questionnaire completion [8].

The second Framingham syncope report [9] noted that 10% of 7814 subjects admitted to at least one syncope spell over a 17-year sampling time. The estimated incidence rate of a first spell was 0.6% per year. However this report contained a sizable minority of patients who had not had a syncope spell, but rather strokes, transient ischemic attacks, and seizures. All diagnoses were established by chart review rather than prospective data collection. The implications of this work remain to be established.

Chen *et al.* [10] performed an extensive community-based study of American adults aged 45 years and older and noted that 19% admitted to at least one lifetime syncope spell. This comes closer to earlier and later estimates.

Recently two groups—in Calgary and Amsterdam—reported remarkably similar results for estimates of community lifetime cumulative incidence. Ganzeboom *et al.* [3] surveyed a semicaptive population of knowledgeable young people (medical students) and found that 39% had fainted at least once by about age 25. Women were almost twice as likely as men to faint (47% vs 24%). The Calgary group recognized the advantages of this population and repeated the study, including almost all first-degree relatives [5]. The oldest parent was 70 years old. Using actuarial analysis this provided an estimate of age-dependent cumulative incidence over all but the last 10–15 years of life. The likelihood of at least one faint was 37% by age 60, and almost all first spells occurred by age 40. In the Calgary study there was no evidence of a second surge of the likelihood of a first faint over 60 years. Taken together, the studies consistently suggest that 40% of people faint at least once in their lives. These results are consistent with several, but not all, of the previous studies.

The most likely reasons for the differences between the estimates include recall error, possible evasion, and discounting of syncope as a medical condition, particularly in childhood. However, it is possible that the differences are real, and they reflect either biological or environmental differences in the populations. For example, African-American blood donors are much less likely to faint than their European contemporaries in the same setting [11].

When does syncope start?

Driscoll *et al.* reported that the age of a "first faint" in a population of children and adolescents under 22 years was highest between ages 15 and 19 years [2]. Although fainting in the very young is well recognized and often termed "reflex anoxic seizures," its incidence is not very well known.

Both Ganzeboom *et al.* [3] and Serletis *et al.* [5] reported very similar age-dependent results in studies of medical students and their families. Vasovagal syncope appears to be quite uncommon before age 8, and the incidence of first faint accelerates rapidly through adolescence. This was true for each of the populations of medical students, their healthy parents, and their siblings. The modal age at first faint—the age at which the largest proportion of people have their first faint—is about 14 years, and the median age of first faint is about 18 years. Males and females begin to faint at the same age. Very few people, about 6%, have a first faint after age 40. Indeed, an early age of onset of syncope is almost pathognomonic of vasovagal syncope. Therefore people in the community who have vasovagal syncope begin fainting at an early age.

Interestingly, patients with vasovagal syncope who are referred for assessment have a very similar age of first onset, with modal and median ages of 14 and 18 years [4]. Also, in this population, there is a second subtle peak of late-onset vasovagal syncope between ages 40 and 60 years, seen particularly in men.

Fainting and the female gender

Societal myths abound that fainting is a female problem, the simple swoon of Victorian romances. Is there truth in this? Serletis *et al.* [5] reported that by age 60, 31% of males and 42% of females had fainted, which is very similar to the proportions reported by Ganzeboom *et al.* [3]. Even more strikingly, although both males and females begin fainting at the same age, the proportion of females who faint reaches an asymptote by about age 30, while the proportion of males who faint reaches its asymptote by about age 50. Therefore, not only are females more likely to faint than males, but young females are particularly more likely to faint than young males.

When do people present for care?

Given that 40% of people faint at least once in their life, why are health care systems not completely swamped with syncope patients? This has been studied in a comparison of community-based and referral-based populations [12].

The referral-based population had a higher median lifetime syncope frequency (1.2 spells/yr vs 0.1 spells/yr), and more subjects began fainting after age 35 (26% vs 6%, $p < 0.0001$). Interestingly, the median frequency of syncope spells in the year preceding referral was higher than that in all previous years (3 spells/yr vs 0.6 spells/yr). The referral-based patient population that started fainting over 35 years presented earlier after their first syncope spell than patients with a younger onset of syncope (median 2.8 yr vs 14.7 yr). From these and similar data it appears that many people tolerate fainting infrequently but present when their syncope frequency intensifies. The earlier presentation of patients who begin to faint over 35 years seems to be due to a much more rapid transit from a benign course, to one with more frequent spells in those who present for medical attention. Interestingly, these data also provide evidence for clustering of syncope: patients do well for many years and then worsen about fivefold. From clinical trials data it appears that many untreated patient populations improve about 80–90% after assessment, in keeping with a transient cluster of syncope lasting months to a few years.

Clinical epidemiology of syncope

The clinical epidemiology of syncope as assessed in medical centers is quite different from its community epidemiology. There are important differences in the prevalence of each cause of syncope, in the age of the patients, in the clinical setting, and importantly for comparative analyses, in the ages reported in studies from different countries.

The proportion of patient visits to family doctors for syncope is not understood very well, except perhaps in the Netherlands. In this regard, Colman et al. [1] reported that about 0.2–0.9% of patient visits were for syncope, and most were for vasovagal syncope [1, review]. Only 10% were referred to specialists. There is an early peak incidence around 15 years for young women (see above) and a later significant rise in visits for both sexes over 65 years. The reason for the increased visits from older patients could be a true increase in community incidence, a concern about a first faint in later years with comorbidities or about the consequences of syncope. Which is true is not known.

The clinical epidemiology of syncope is better understood in the emergency department environment. We now have quite detailed insights into the composition of syncope patients. The proportion of emergency room visits due to syncope is about 1% in Italy, France, and the United States. Ammirati et al. studied 195 syncope patients in the emergency wards of nine community hospitals around Rome [13]. They had a mean age of 63 years, and 44% were men. About 34% had vasovagal syncope and another 2% had carotid sinus syncope. Cardiac syncope—mainly due to arrhythmias—occurred in 21% and orthostatic hypotension in 6%. About 14% were deemed to have seizures or cerebrovascular disease (not truly syncope syndromes), 6% had pseudosyncope, and 18% had eluded diagnosis. Therefore in contrast to the general population, Roman syncope patients are older, have more cardiovascular disease and more arrhythmias, and are more likely to have orthostatic hypotension.

Blanc *et al.* studied 454 patients with syncope in Brest, with mean age 57 years, of whom 43% were men [14]. A cause of syncope was found in 76%. The most common diagnosis was vasovagal syncope (44%), and 1–2% each had causes such as cough syncope, carotid syncope, and sneeze syncope. Cardiac arrhythmias were found in 8%, and a further 12% were thought to have nonsyncope syndromes, such as hypoglycemia. Again, Brest syncope patients are older and have more cardiac arrhythmias than the community population probably has.

Shen *et al.* used a dedicated syncope unit to study syncope epidemiology in a midwestern American emergency ward [15]. There were 52 patients with mean age 64 years, and 49% were men. Of these, 52% had vasovagal syncope, 18% eluded diagnosis, 12% carotid sinus syncope, 6% cardiac syncope, and 10% orthostatic syncope or drug effects.

These studies are generally similar. Overall, syncope patients in emergency wards are older, with a mean age of about 60 years. About 50% probably have a manifestation of vasovagal syncope, 5–20% have a form of cardiac syncope, perhaps 5% each have carotid sinus syncope or orthostatic hypotension, and there is a persistent minority of 10–20% with nonsyncope syndromes also referred to assessment. Therefore the emergency department patient with syncope is an older person who has several potential causes other than vasovagal syncope.

Syncope in the older patient

There are few community-based studies of syncope in the elderly, but there is a voluminous literature on syncope in the aged patient. In a clinical epidemiology report, Lipsitz *et al.* [16] studied 711 nursing home residents and found a yearly incidence of 6% and a 2-year recurrence rate of 30%. The patients tended to be the frail elderly with numerous competing diagnoses and risk factors. Only 3% of the spells were thought to be due to typical vasovagal syncope.

Epidemiology-based decision making

The major competing diagnoses for TLOC are syncope and epileptic seizures, although less common possibilities such as narcolepsy, cataplexy, and pseudoseizures and pseudosyncope should be remembered. The lifetime prevalence of generalized seizures due to epilepsy is 0.4–0.7%, based on estimates derived from Britain and China [17, 18]. In contrast, the lifetime prevalence of syncope appears to be much higher.

The statistical problem becomes clear. With community lifetime cumulative incidences of 40% for syncope and 0.4% for epileptic seizures, any diagnostic tool will either overinclude syncope patients or underinclude patients with epileptic seizures. Indeed, about 25% of patients with a diagnosis of epilepsy may truly have syncope.

Where to go from here?

Epidemiology describes that which we hope to modify. Several topics need to be addressed. First, we still know relatively little about the natural history of vasovagal syncope, and our risk stratification tools are blunt. Are there truly clusters of syncope, and if so, how often do they occur and how long do they last? What are the predictors of entering and exiting a cluster?

Second, we know relatively little about the community-based epidemiology of syncope. Is there truly a late surge of syncope "first presentations" after 65 years, or is the surge seen in clinics only a reflection of referral bias? If there is a surge, what are the etiologies of the syncope? What are the relative proportions of the different syndromes in family doctors' offices compared to specialty clinics, and are there predictors of referrals of high-risk patients? What explains the difference in mean ages in syncope populations in North America and Europe?

Third, we need to develop methodologies for ascertaining diagnoses that are simple, inexpensive, and noninvasive. Although both tilt-table tests and implantable loop recorders would be difficult to use in epidemiologic studies, the disproportionate population sizes of the different diagnostic entities will cause problems with predictive values, and therefore more than a simple questionnaire may need to be used [19, 20]. New diagnostic strategies are needed.

References

1 Colman N, Nahm K, Ganzeboom KS, *et al*. Epidemiology of reflex syncope. *Clin Auton Res* 2004;**14**(suppl 1):9–17.

2 Driscoll DJ, Jacobsen SJ, Porter CJ, Wollan PC. Syncope in children and adolescents. *J Am Coll Cardiol* 1997;**29**:1039–45.

3 Ganzeboom KS, Colman N, Reitsma JB, Shen WK, Wieling W. Prevalence and triggers of syncope in medical students. *Am J Cardiol* 2003;**91**:1006–8.

4 Koshman ML, Ritchie D; Investigators of the Syncope Symptom Study and the Prevention of Syncope Trial. Age of first faint in patients with vasovagal syncope. *J Cardiovasc Electrophysiol* 2006;**17**(1):49–54.

5 Serletis A, Rose S, Sheldon AG, Sheldon RS. Vasovagal syncope in medical students and their first-degree relatives. *Eur Heart J* 2006;**27**(16):1965–70.

6 Dermksian G, Lamb LE. Syncope in a population of healthy young adults. *J Am Med Assoc* 1958;**168**:1200–7.

7 Savage DD, Corwin L, McGee DL, *et al*. Epidemiologic features of isolated syncope: the Framingham study. *Stroke* 1985;**16**:626–9.

8 Barry D. Differential recall bias and spurious associations in case/control studies. *Stat Med* 1996;**15**:2603–16.

9 Soteriades ES, Evans JC, Larson MG, *et al.* Incidence and prognosis of syncope. *N Engl J Med* 2002;**347**(12):878–85.

10 Chen LY, Shen WK, Mahoney DW, Jacobsen SJ, Rodeheffer RJ. Prevalence of syncope in a population aged more than 45 years. *Am J Med* 2006;**119**(12):1088.e1–7.

11 Newman BH. Vasovagal reactions in high school student: findings relative to race, risk factor synergism, female sex, and non-high school participants. *Transfusion* 2002;**42**:1557–60.

12 Sheldon RS, Sheldon AG, Serletis A, *et al.*; for the Investigators of the Prevention of Syncope Study. Worsening of symptoms before presentation with vasovagal syncope. *J Cardiovasc Electrophysiol*, 2007. In press.

13 Ammirati F, Colivicchi F, Santini M; on behalf of the Investigators of the OESIL Study Diagnosing syncope in clinical practice. Implementation of a simplified diagnostic algorithm in a multicenter prospective trial—the OESIL 2 Study (Osservatorio Epidemiologico della Sincope nel Lazio). *Eur Heart J* 2000;**21**:935–40.

14 Blanc JJ, L'Her C, Touiza A, Garo B, L'Her E, Mansourati J. Prospective evaluation and outcome of patients admitted for syncope over a 1 year period. *Eur Heart J* 2002;**23**:815–20.

15 Shen WK, Decker WW, Smars PA, *et al.* Syncope Evaluation in the Emergency Department Study (SEEDS): a multidisciplinary approach to syncope management. *Circulation* 2004;**110**(24):3636–45.

16 Lipsitz LA, Pluchino FC, Wei JY, Rowe JW. Syncope in an elderly institutionalized population: prevalence, incidence and associated risk. *Q J Med* 1985;**55**:45–54.

17 Macdonald BK, Cockerel OC, Sander JWAS, Shorvon SD. The incidence and lifetime prevalence of lifetime neurologic disorders in a prospective community-based study in the UK. *Brain* 2000;**123**:665–76.

18 Kwan P, Sander JW. The natural history of epilepsy: an epidemiological view. *J Neurol Neurosurg Psychiatry* 2004;**75**:1376–81.

19 Sheldon R, Rose S, Ritchie D, *et al.* Historical criteria that distinguish syncope from seizures. *J Am Coll Cardiol* 2002;**40**:142–8.

20 Sheldon R, Rose S, Ritchie D, Koshman ML, Connolly S, Frenneaux M. Historical diagnostic criteria for vasovagal syncope in the absence of structural heart disease. *Eur Heart J* 2006;**27**:344–50.

CHAPTER 3

Pathophysiology of syncope: postural, neurally-mediated, and arrhythmic

W Wieling

Introduction

Syncope is a symptom characterized by self-limited loss of consciousness due to transient global cerebral hypoperfusion. The underlying mechanism is most often a fall in systemic blood pressure. Other less common causes include transient diminution of ambient oxygen tension.

Syncope usually occurs when the victim is in the upright position. In some individuals, syncope may be triggered by movement from the seated or supine position to the upright posture (so-called postural or "orthostatic" faints). In other instances the hypotension may be the result of neurally-mediated reflex disturbances in blood pressure control (e.g., vasovagal faint) or the transient reduction of cardiac output (CO) (mainly the result of arrhythmias). Recent insights that further our understanding of postural, neurally-mediated, and arrhythmic syncope will be reviewed.

Physiology of upright posture

When humans stand up, 500–1000 mL of blood is transferred from the chest to the distensible venous system below the diaphragm. Up to 50% of the total shift occurs within the first 10 seconds. Most of this pooled blood is contained within the large deep veins of the legs [1]. Pooling in the splanchnic area during actual orthostasis (standing/head-up tilting) seems to be more important than that previously reported in studies using simulated orthostasis by applying lower body negative pressure [2].

Mechanical factors are important in opposing gravitational pooling of blood. Leg crossing and contraction of leg and abdominal muscles have been shown to be beneficial to prevent orthostatic and vasovagal faints [3]. Another option is to enhance the thoracoabdominal pump effect by inspiration through a narrow lumen or predetermined resistance device (impedance threshold device, ITD) that acts as a resistance [4]. In the case of the ITD, the forced increase in negative intrathoracic pressure during inspiration acts to enhance

Syncope and Transient Loss of Consciousness, 1st edition. Edited by David G Benditt *et al.*
© 2007 Blackwell Publishing, ISBN: 978-1-4051-7625-5.

venous return to the central circulation and at the same time improve the gradient for blood flow across the cerebral circulation.

The instantaneous and fast venous pooling of blood on arising results in a rapid diminution of the central blood volume. Unless compensatory adjustments are promptly instituted, arterial pressure falls and the subject faints or develops symptoms of a near faint (e.g., light-headedness and temporary diminished vision). The arterial (especially carotid) baroreceptor control of sympathetic vasomotor tone of resistance and splanchnic capacitance vessels is the most important component in the maintenance of postural normotension in humans [1].

The adjustment to upright posture (orthostatic adjustment) may reasonably be classified into three phases: *an initial response* (first 30 s), *an early phase of stabilization* (1–2 min upright), and *prolonged orthostasis* (>5 min upright). This classification is both appropriate from the physiological perspective and of direct clinical relevance [1]. The first (initial) phase corresponds to immediate complaints of presyncope and syncope upon arising suddenly after prolonged supine rest or after arising from the squatted position [5]. The second (early) phase accounts for blood pressure measurements commonly used to assess orthostatic hypotension in the office or bedside. Depending on the clinical setting, orthostatic hypotension will be detected in 50–100% of the patients with autonomic disturbances within 3 minutes in the upright posture [6]. The third phase corresponds with delayed orthostatic hypotension, such as in the postural tachycardia syndrome and susceptibility to vasovagal fainting [6, 7].

Neurally-mediated syncope

Syncope has a bimodal temporal distribution, with a first peak in the teenagers, adolescents, and young adults and a second peak in subjects >70 years. In young patients almost all instances of syncope are neural reflex mediated and most occur in the upright posture (here termed "orthostatic vasovagal syncope").

Orthostatic vasovagal fainting usually occurs when the CO for any reason has decreased by about 50% [1]. The final classical event as observed during tilt-table testing in young subjects is vasodilatation and a distinct vagally-mediated bradycardia with a rapid fall in blood pressure [7]. A marked fall in stroke volume (SV) and cardiac output (CO) occurs in elderly patients prior to the actual faint during tilt-table testing. Age-related impairments in early diastolic ventricular filling and thereby in SV induced by preload reduction can play an important role in this pronounced CO decrease [7]. In the elderly, the reflex bradycardia component during presyncope is far less pronounced than in the young, and the fall in systemic blood pressure tends to be much more gradual [7]. This difference can be attributed to an attenuated vagal heart rate control in the elderly. However, in contrast to the attenuated bradycardic response during tilt-table-testing-induced vasovagal syncope, a marked bradycardia and prolonged asystole are common observations in elderly subjects presumed to have vasovagal syncope on clinical grounds when studied with an implantable loop recorder [8]. At present this discrepancy is hard to explain [7], but important inasmuch as it diminishes utility of tilt-table testing for predicting the mode of subsequent spontaneous neurally-mediated faints.

Arrhythmic syncope

The influence of cardiac arrhythmias on systemic blood pressure is dependent on the effect of the arrhythmia on CO and the effectiveness of the baroreflex-mediated sympathetic vasomotor counterregulation. The classical example of arrhythmic syncope is the so-called Stokes–Adams attack, occurring as a result of intermittent heart block. Prominent facial flushing upon regaining consciousness after an episode of transient loss of consciousness is thought to be pathognomonic for a Stokes–Adams attack. However, a recent study showed that this widely accepted "fact" is not always correct. When blood pressure recovers rapidly on return to the supine posture, a pronounced facial flush also occurs in patients with vasovagal syncope (Figure 3.1). The facial flush is caused by well-oxygenated blood that is pumped into a constricted arteriolar bed.

The influence of tachyarrhythmias on systemic blood pressure is complex. A marked abrupt blood pressure decrease starting immediately after the onset of a supraventricular tachycardia (SVT) has been described in patients with normal hearts. The nadir is in the first 10 seconds and a gradual recovery occurs within 30 seconds despite the persistent tachycardia [10]. In the upright posture the changes are more prominent. Sudden atrial distension and vigorous atrial contraction against closed atrioventricular valves with reflex vasodilatation have been postulated to underlie the initial transient fall in blood pressure [10]. In elderly patients with cardiac disease, additional factors may aggravate susceptibility to hypotension. In particular, CO can be threatened by SVT (in particular atrial fibrillation), because the time available to adequately fill the ventricle (especially in the setting of age-related diastolic dysfunction) is shortened and may be inadequate to maintain an adequate CO.

In patients with sustained ventricular tachycardia (VT), an arrhythmia that tends to be associated with underlying left ventricular disease, CO is further diminished from baseline value, thereby accounting for low systemic blood pressure. The role of subsequent reflex adjustments in this setting is largely unknown. However, not all VT cause hypotension (e.g., most idiopathic left ventricular fascicular tachycardias and right ventricular outflow tract tachycardias). The observation that some patients maintain a good blood pressure during VT (even in the setting of heart disease) strongly suggests that peripheral factors are important in determining hemodynamic consequences of the tachyarrhythmia.

In patients with conditions such as hypertrophic cardiomyopathy or aortic stenosis, both SVT and VT may cause cardiac syncope. However, neurally-mediated reflex syncope is also common in these patients. Reflex syncope in these patients is thought to be elicited by triggers from the hypertrophic heart itself, presumably by ventricular and atrial mechanoreceptors. The presence of

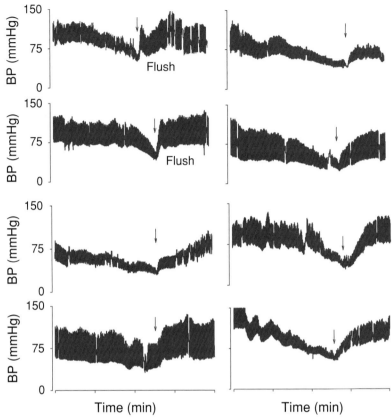

Figure 3.1 Continuous finger blood pressure recordings during tilt-induced faints. Arrows indicate tilt to horizontal. Pronounced flushing was observed in the patients in the upper-left panels. The presence of facial flushing was associated with a rapid return to physiological blood pressure levels, suggesting that the faints in these two patients were CO mediated. (Taken with permission from [9].)

abnormal or exaggerated reflex responses may aggravate the adverse hemodynamic impact of a concomitant arrhythmia.

Conclusion

Understanding of the mechanisms of hypotension causing syncope remains incomplete. Nevertheless, recent studies have provided valuable insights into the pathophysiology of certain most common causes of syncope. Consideration of these mechanisms is of value in order to address treatment of orthostatic and neurally-mediated reflex faints in particular and for better understanding the range of hemodynamic responses to cardiac arrhythmias observed in clinical practice.

References

1 Wieling W, van Lieshout JJ. Maintenance of postural normotension in humans. In: Low P (ed.), *Auton Disord*, 2007. In press.
2 Taneja I, Moran C, Medow MS, *et al.* Differential effects of lower body negative pressure and upright tilt on splanchnic blood volume. *Am J Physiol (Heart Circ Physiol)* 2007;**292**:H420–6.
3 Krediet CTP, de Bruin IG, Ganzeboom KS, *et al.* Leg crossing, muscle tensing, squatting, and the crash position are effective against vasovagal reactions solely through increases in cardiac output. *J Appl Physiol* 2005;**99**:1697–703.
4 Thijs RD, Wieling W, Aardweg JG, *et al.* Respiratory countermaneuvers in autonomic failure. *Neurology*, 2007. In press.
5 Wieling W, Krediet CTP, van Dijk N, *et al.* Initial hypotension: review of a forgotten condition. *Clin Sci* 2007;**112**:157–65.
6 Gibbons CH, Freeman R. Delayed orthostatic hypotension. *Neurology* 2006;**67**:28–32.
7 Verheyden B, Gisolf J, Beckers F, *et al.* Sublingual nitroglycerine provokes distinct age-related vasovagal responses during routine tilt testing. *Clin Sci*, 2007. In press.
8 Brignole M, Sutton R, Wieling W, *et al.* Analysis of rhythm variation during spontaneous cardioinhibitory neurally-mediated syncope: implications for RDR pacing optimization. An ISSUE 2 substudy. *Europace* 2007;**9**:305–11.
9 Wieling W, Krediet CTP, Wilde AA. Flush after syncope: not always an arrhythmia. *J Cardiovasc Electrophysiol* 2006;**17**:804–5.
10 Ravazi M, Luria DM, Jahangir A, *et al.* Acute blood pressure changes after the onset of atrioventricular nodal reentrant tachycardia: a time-course analysis. *J Cardiovasc Electrophysiol* 2005;**16**:1037–40.

CHAPTER 4

Cerebral perfusion in syncope

J Gert van Dijk, Roland D Thijs

Introduction

In syncope, the systemic circulation fails to keep cardiac output and/or blood pressure within normal bounds, causing a decrease in cerebral blood flow (CBF) leading to loss of consciousness. CBF is complicated by the enclosure of the brain in the inflexible skull. An increase in the volume of brain, the cerebrospinal fluid, or its blood volume must be compensated by a decrease in volume of the rest of the skull contents, or intracranial pressure will rise, compromising perfusion.

CBF cannot be measured directly, but the flow velocity of the middle cerebral artery can be measured with transcranial Doppler devices (TCD). Flow velocity is a good measure of flow, provided that flow is laminar and the vessel diameter stays the same [1], which luckily is the case for vessels of this magnitude over a wide range of mean arterial pressure (MAP) and CO_2 levels.

This chapter first briefly reviews factors affecting CBF and then discusses specific features in reflex syncope and autonomic failure, and it ends with conditions in which CBF is compromised separate from the systemic circulation.

Cerebral perfusion

MAP is a major determinant of CBF. However, CBF does not simply follow fluctuations in MAP, but remains stable over a wide arterial pressure range (about 60–160 mmHg) due to cerebral autoregulation. If MAP falls below the lower limit of autoregulation, CBF does follow MAP; this sudden failure is readily apparent from the electroencephalogram (EEG) in tilt-induced syncope: the EEG stays normal for a long time, while MAP decreases, but when it does change, slow waves, a flat EEG, and unconsciousness all develop in seconds. The mechanisms of autoregulation are not entirely clear, but apparently depend for the most part on muscle fibers in small arterial walls functioning without neural supervision and, to a lesser extent, if at all, on sympathetically driven influences.

Syncope and Transient Loss of Consciousness, 1st edition. Edited by David G Benditt *et al.*
© 2007 Blackwell Publishing, ISBN: 978-1-4051-7625-5.

Obviously, CBF depends on all factors affecting perfusion besides arterial pressure. For most organs, perfusion pressure is the difference between arterial and venous pressure, but in the brain, tissue pressure (intracranial pressure) can add significantly to the equation. Perfusion pressure in the brain is, therefore, often calculated as the difference between arterial and intracranial pressures. Active tension in the vessel wall plays a role in the "critical closing pressure": the pressure in the lumen that is just too low to keep it open against pressures tending to close it, i.e., wall tension and intracranial pressure.

Wall tension is the agent of autoregulation: when MAP decreases, tension is decreased in small arterioles that open up to allow more flow. CO_2 is important here, as hypocapnia has a potent vasoconstrictor effect. Hyperventilation therefore tends to decrease CBF, but, as often is the case in CBF physiology, factors interact: selective increase of inspiratory ventilatory effort activates the respiratory pump and thereby augments venous return. MAP increases as a result, and this may be helpful in combating hypotension in autonomic failure [2, 3]. These respiratory efforts will be most helpful when inspiratory pressures can become lower without lowering CO_2, as hyperventilation causes cerebral vasoconstriction and hypotension in autonomic failure.

Cerebral perfusion in reflex syncope

In neurally-mediated reflex syncope, cardioinhibition, vasodilatation, or both, impair the systemic circulation. A typical TCD finding just before syncope is normal systolic and decreased diastolic flow velocity. The resulting change in pulsatility index (PI) was initially interpreted to suggest a paradoxical vasoconstriction, but more recent analyses suggest that PI is not an appropriate indicator of flow resistance in this context. Instead, resistance estimates based on the ratio of blood pressure and flow velocity suggested low resistance; i.e., autoregulation was doing its best to keep CBF going [4]. Similar conclusions were drawn by others [5, 6]. An apparent failure of autoregulation was probably due to MAP falling below the autoregulation range [5]. The preferential decrease of diastolic flow was explained through blood pressure becoming so low that some vessels collapsed in diastole, as their critical closing pressure was passed [6].

Cerebral perfusion in autonomic failure

In autonomic failure, blood pressure decreases in the upright position because the sympathetic system fails to prevent blood pooling in the lower parts of the body. As cerebral autoregulation is, in part, thought to be mediated through the sympathetic system, it might also be affected. Clinical experience, however, suggests that autonomic failure patients can remain conscious at extremely low MAP values, suggesting that autoregulation remains intact for the most part.

Several authors investigated autoregulation by examining the relationship between paired MAP and flow velocity measurements: if autoregulation works, there should be no relationship, because flow velocity should remain stable in spite of changing MAP. If velocity does vary with MAP, the relationship would signify defective autoregulation. Some studies suggested normal autoregulation [7, 8], whereas others pointed to defective autoregulation [9, 10]. There are several differences in methods and possibly in patient groups, making it impossible to explain the discrepancy in results without further study.

Local cerebral perfusion problems

As noted above, a failure of the systemic circulation is almost always the cause of syncope (i.e., a drop in systemic pressure below the lower limits of autoregulation). However, on rare occasions the cerebral circulation may itself be to blame for several less well-defined attacks of unconsciousness. For instance, a transient ischemic attack of one carotid artery does not normally cause unconsciousness, but it can do so when the remaining vessels are already compromised or completely occluded. By way of another example, high intrathoracic pressure can compromise CBF; this apparently occurs in cough syncope, where venous cerebral pressure increases so much that it counteracts arterial pressure, stopping cerebral perfusion; a reflex syncope is probably also involved, and in individual patients, their respective contributions are unknown. A similar mechanism may explain unconsciousness in the "blue breath-holding spells" of toddlers caught in an expiratory Valsalva-like spasm. Sudden increases in intracranial pressure can also cause sudden unconsciousness: in subarachnoid hemorrhage, the sudden influx of arterial blood in the subarachnoid space increases intracranial pressure, lowering perfusion pressure.

Conclusion

By definition, the occurrence of transient loss of consciousness in syncope is the result of diminished CBF. The primary, but not exclusive, cause of diminished CBF is a self-limited fall in systemic blood pressure. The factors that control CBF are complex as well as the principal contributors have been summarized here. It should be recognized, however, that disease states and concomitant medications may further modify CBF control and consequent susceptibility to syncope.

References

1 van Lieshout JJ, Wieling W, Karemaker JM, Secher NH. Syncope, cerebral perfusion, and oxygenation. *J Appl Physiol* 2003;**94**:833–48.
2 Melby DP, Lu F, Sakaguchi S, Zook M, Benditt DG. Increased impedance to inspiration ameliorates hemodynamic changes associated with movement to upright posture in orthostatic hypotension: a randomized blinded pilot study. *Heart Rhythm* 2007;**4**:128–35.
3 Thijs RD, Wieling W, Aardweg JG, van Dijk JG. Respiratory countermaneuvers in autonomic failure. *Neurology*, 2007. In press.
4 Schondorf R, Benoit J, Wein T. Cerebrovascular and cardiovascular measurements during neurally mediated syncope induced by head-up tilt. *Stroke* 1997;**28**:1564–8.

5 Carey BJ, Manktelow BN, Panerai RB, Potter JF. Cerebral autoregulatory responses to head-up tilt in normal subjects and patients with recurrent vasovagal syncope. *Circulation* 2001;**104**:898–902.

6 Carey BJ, Eames PJ, Panerai RB, Potter JF. Carbon dioxide, critical closing pressure and cerebral haemodynamics prior to vasovagal syncope in humans. *Clin Sci* 2001;**101**:351–8.

7 Bondar R, Dunphy PT, Moradshahi P, *et al.* Cerebrovascular and cardiovascular responses to graded tilt in patients with autonomic failure. *Stroke* 1997;**28**:1677–85.

8 Horowitz DR, Kaufman H. Autoregulatory cerebral vasodilation occurs during orthostatic hypotension in patients with autonomic failure. *Clin Auton Res* 2001;**11**:363–7.

9 Novak V, Novak P, Spies JM, Low PA. Autoregulation of cerebral blood flow in orthostatic hypotension. *Stroke* 1998;**29**;104–11.

10 Claydon VE, Hainsworth R. Cerebral autoregulation during orthostatic stress in healthy controls and in patients with posturally related syncope. *Clin Auton Res* 2003;**13**:321–9.

CHAPTER 5

Risk stratification—impact on diagnostic strategy

Brian Olshansky

An aborted cardiac arrest can resemble syncope. Syncope can therefore appear the same as sudden death except that the patient wakes up [1]. Clearly, then, identifying the patient with transient loss of consciousness at high risk of sudden and total mortality is critical.

Are syncope patients at risk of dying?

Syncope predicted mortality in the Framingham study [2]. Those diagnosed with "cardiac syncope" were at greater risk of dying. Patients with syncope of unknown cause and syncope due to a presumed neurologic cause (although it is uncertain what the authors meant by this latter term) were at increased risk, and those with vasovagal causes for syncope were not. Similarly, in a 5-year follow-up of patients hospitalized for syncope [3] and in patients presenting to an emergency department [4], the mortality rate was highest for those with a cardiac syncope. These data, however, do not indicate that syncope is an independent risk factor for mortality even in patients with diagnosed heart disease.

Underlying comorbidities may be the reason patients with syncope appear to be at higher risk of sudden death. In one report [5], patients with and without syncope had similar rates of 1-year overall and cardiac mortality. Underlying cardiac disease, not syncope, predicted mortality.

High-risk cardiac conditions can cause syncope

The presence of heart disease does not necessarily indicate that syncope is cardiac or even life threatening [6]. Potentially malignant cardiovascular conditions that can explain syncope include:

1 hemodynamic impairment from poor ventricular function or poor cardiovascular adjustment to physical stressors;

2 obstruction to cardiac output with an apparent dysfunctional reflex response;

Syncope and Transient Loss of Consciousness, 1st edition. Edited by David G Benditt *et al.*
© 2007 Blackwell Publishing, ISBN: 978-1-4051-7625-5.

3 poorly tolerated ventricular tachycardia due to various conditions (cardiomyopathies, infiltrative diseases, arrhythmogenic right ventricular cardiomyopathy, hypertrophic cardiomyopathy, long QT-interval syndrome, congenital heart diseases, and various channelopathies);

4 poorly tolerated supraventricular arrhythmias; and

5 episodic asystole.

From a retrospective database, Middlekauff *et al.* [7] reported that 12% of 491 functional class III–IV patients (mean left ventricular ejection fraction 0.20) had syncope. The 1-year sudden death rate was 45% in syncope patients versus 12% in patients without syncope ($p < 0.00001$). These data are supported by a recent subanalysis of the Sudden Cardiac Death in Heart Failure Trial (SCD-HeFT) data in which heart failure patients with syncope had a higher mortality than those without syncope [8].

Is electrophysiology testing predictive?

Electrophysiology (EP) testing may be diagnostic [9] and may risk-stratify but the predictive value is only 'fair', and its value is primarily for patients already at highest risk (i.e., those with poor ejection fraction, coronary artery disease, and heart failure). EP testing predicts risk for total and cardiac mortality and risk for implantable cardioverter-defibrillator (ICD) shocks in patients with structural heart disease who have syncope or ventricular tachycardia [10, 11]. EP testing has little value for many conditions, including the long QT-interval syndrome, Brugada syndrome, sarcoidosis, arrhythmogenic right ventricular cardiomyopathy, dilated cardiomyopathy, and hypertrophic cardiomyopathy.

Patients with a positive EP test and structural heart disease are at great risk whether they present with syncope, ventricular tachycardia, or ventricular fibrillation [12]. Patients with heart disease and inducible ventricular tachyarrhythmias at EP study, who undergo ICD implant, have similar outcomes whether they have syncope or ventricular tachycardia [13].

Use of EP testing has become even more limited by virtue of the broad guidelines advocating use of ICDs for primary prevention in patients with impaired ventricular function regardless of syncope. Patients now considered for EP testing include those who have structural heart disease or bundle branch block, but do not otherwise have an indication for an ICD. The role for the signal-averaged electrocardiogram (ECG) or for use of T-wave alternans and other noninvasive testing is uncertain.

ICD in heart failure patients with syncope—do they help?

Patients with syncope and dilated cardiomyopathy undergoing ICD implants [14] have a similar risk of mortality and ICD shocks, compared with patients who have had prior cardiac arrest. Data from SCD-HeFT support the notion that ICD discharges are common in syncope patients with cardiomyopathy and heart failure, but compared with placebo, ICDs do not improve survival in syncope patients [8].

An approach to evaluating syncope

Cardiovascular conditions as cause for syncope should be considered for all syncope patients. The evaluation should be based on evidence derived from the history and physical examination. Any ensuing diagnostic evaluation is derived from the patient's clinical presentation and the level of suspicion of heart disease. An ECG is warranted in all patients (including those in whom other non-syncope causes of transient loss of consciousness, such as 'seizures', are being contemplated as the diagnosis), but otherwise there is no evidence to support generalized use of more involved routine testing. Predictors of poor outcomes include evidence for heart disease, including an abnormal ECG [15].

New approaches to decision making and risk stratification

New approaches to risk stratification have been tested in acute settings. Osservatorio Epidemiologico della Sincope nel Lazio (OESIL), OESIL 2, the San Francisco Syncope Rule (SFSR), and other standardized approaches attempt to improve the chance of achieving a diagnosis and predicting outcomes [16–18]. The OESIL risk score (age >65 yr; history of cardiovascular disease, syncope without prodrome, and an abnormal ECG) may not be sensitive or specific enough. Other approaches that are being tested (e.g., the ROSE trial [19]) include use of the American College of Emergency Physicians (ACEP) clinical policy to identify patients with cardiac cause for syncope [20]. ACEP level B recommendations have a high sensitivity and are relatively specific to diagnose cardiac syncope in the emergency department.

Conclusion

It is important to distinguish which patient with syncope is at high risk of death. Risk stratification impacts diagnostic strategy and is best accomplished by utilizing effective strategies that can identify presence of cardiovascular risk. The starting point is a careful and perhaps standardized evaluation (history, physical examination, and ECG). Any subsequent invasive or noninvasive testing is based on this initial evaluation. No specific, more involved diagnostic strategy has been shown to be better than this for the syncope patient. As such, syncope evaluation remains at a crossroad [21], as it is not exactly clear for whom the bell tolls [22]. Identifying patient with transient loss of consciousness at high risk of death remains a challenge.

References

1 Olshansky B. Is syncope the same thing as sudden death except that you wake up? *J Cardiovasc Electrophysiol* 1997;**8**(10):1098–101.

2 Soteriades ES, Evans JC, Larson MG, *et al.* Incidence and prognosis of syncope. *N Engl J Med* 2002;**347**(12):878–85.

3 Racco F, Sconocchini C, Alesi C, *et al.* Long-term follow-up after syncope: a group of 183 patients observed for 5 years. *Minerva Cardioangiol* 2000;**48**(3):69–78.

4 Schillinger M, Mullner M, Meron G, *et al.* Causes and outcome of syncope. *Wien Klin Wochenschr* 1999;**111**(13):512–16.

5 Kapoor WN, Hanusa BH. Is syncope a risk factor for poor outcomes? Comparison of patients with and without syncope. *Am J Med* 1996;**100**(6):646–55.

6 Alboni P, Brignole M, Menozzi C, *et al.* Diagnostic value of history in patients with syncope with or without heart disease. *J Am Coll Cardiol* 2001;**37**(7):1921–8.

7 Middlekauff HR, Stevenson WG, Saxon LA. Prognosis after syncope: impact of left ventricular function. *Am Heart J* 1993;**125**(1):121–7.

8 Olshansky B, Poole JE, Johnson GW, *et al.* Syncope predicts outcome of cardiomyopathy patients—analysis of the SCD-HeFT Trial. *Circulation* 2005;**12**:II454.

9 Olshansky B, Mazuz M, Martins JB. Significance of inducible tachycardia in patients with syncope of unknown origin: a long-term follow-up. *J Am Coll Cardiol* 1985;**5**(2, pt 1): 216–23.

10 Pires LA, May LM, Ravi S, *et al.* Comparison of event rates and survival in patients with unexplained syncope without documented ventricular tachyarrhythmias versus patients with documented sustained ventricular tachyarrhythmias both treated with implantable cardioverter-defibrillators. *Am J Cardiol* 2000;**85**(6):725–8.

11 Andrews NP, Fogel RI, Pelargonio G, *et al.* Implantable defibrillator event rates in patients with unexplained syncope and inducible sustained ventricular tachyarrhythmias: a comparison with patients known to have sustained ventricular tachycardia. *J Am Coll Cardiol* 1999;**34**(7):2023–30.

12 Olshansky B, Hahn EA, Hartz VL, *et al.*; ESVEM Investigators. Clinical significance of syncope in the electrophysiologic study versus electrocardiographic monitoring (ESVEM) trial. *Am Heart J* 1999;**137**(5):878–86.

13 Steinberg JS, Beckman K, Greene HL, *et al.* Follow-up of patients with unexplained syncope and inducible ventricular tachyarrhythmias: analysis of the AVID registry and an AVID substudy. Antiarrhythmics versus implantable defibrillators. *J Cardiovasc Electrophysiol* 2001;**12**(9):996–1001.

14 Knight BP, Goyal R, Pelosi F, *et al.* Outcome of patients with nonischemic dilated cardiomyopathy and unexplained syncope treated with an implantable defibrillator. *J Am Coll Cardiol* 1999;**33**(7):1964–70.

15 Martin TP, Hanusa BH, Kapoor WN. Risk stratification of patients with syncope. *Ann Emerg Med* 1997;**29**(4):459–66.

16 Ammirati F, Colivicchi F, Minardi G, *et al.* The management of syncope in the hospital: the OESIL Study (Osservatorio Epidemiologico della Sincope nel Lazio). *G Ital Cardiol* 1999;**29**(5):533–9.

17 Colivicchi F, Ammirati F, Melina D, *et al.* Development and prospective validation of a risk stratification system for patients with syncope in the emergency department: the OESIL risk score. *Eur Heart J* 2003;**24**(9):811–19.

18 Quinn JV, Stiell IG, McDermott DA, *et al.* The San Francisco syncope rule vs physician judgment and decision making. *Am J Emerg Med* 2005;**23**(6):782–6.

19 Reed MJ, Newby DE, Coull AJ, *et al.* The risk stratification of syncope in the emergency department (ROSE) pilot study: a comparison of existing syncope guidelines. *Emerg Med J* 2007;**24**(4):270–5.

20 Elesber AA, Decker WW, Smars PA, *et al*. Impact of the application of the American College of Emergency Physicians recommendations for the admission of patients with syncope on a retrospectively studied population presenting to the emergency department. *Am Heart J* 2005;**149**(5):826–31.

21 Olshansky B. Syncope evaluation at a crossroad: for which patients? *Circulation* 2001;**104**(1):7–8.

22 Olshansky B. For whom does the bell toll? *J Cardiovasc Electrophysiol* 2001;**12**(9):1002–3.

PART 2

Clinical evaluation strategies

CHAPTER 6

Value and limitations of clinical history in assessing cause of syncope

Paolo Alboni, Maurizio Dinelli

If obtained with care and in sufficient detail by an experienced clinician, the medical history alone may be sufficient to provide a diagnosis of the cause of syncope. In other instances, even if not definitively pointing to the cause, historical features may guide the subsequent evaluation strategy. Table 6.1 lists how to use the history and physical findings in suggesting various syncope etiologies [1].

Since the publication of the 2004 ESC Syncope Guidelines, a number of contributions have been made to the literature that alter our concept of the role of history taking in the assessment of the transient loss of consciousness (TLOC)/syncope patient. However, in regard to the real importance of the medical history, they do not substantially change the ESC task force recommendations. These new contributions primarily deal with neurally-mediated reflex syncope, syncope during sleep, syncope in older subjects, and laughter-induced syncope.

New insights regarding the value of history in subjects with neurally-mediated reflex syncope are reported in Chapter 8. Here, we discuss a few other conditions in which concepts have been changing.

Syncope during sleep

Loss of consciousness in the supine position is unusual in syncope and is generally considered an expression of epilepsy or cardiac syncope (i.e., a severe arrhythmia). Recently, a new clinical entity defined as "sleep syncope" has been described [2, 3]. It has been defined as loss of consciousness in a nonintoxicated adult, occurring during the normal hours of sleeping. Most of the subjects are middle-age women. All gave a history of waking from sleep with abdominal discomfort, nausea, or the urge to defecate followed by loss of consciousness. In some subjects syncope occurred in bed, whereas in others while

Syncope and Transient Loss of Consciousness, 1st edition. Edited by David G Benditt *et al.*
© 2007 Blackwell Publishing, ISBN: 978-1-4051-7625-5.

Table 6.1 2004 ESC Syncope Guidelines: clinical features suggestive of specific causes of loss of consciousness.

Neurally-mediated syncope
  Absence of cardiological disease
  Long history of syncope
  After sudden unexpected unpleasant sight, sound, smell, or pain
  Prolonged standing, or crowded and hot places
  Nausea and vomiting associated with syncope
  During the meal or in the absorptive state after a meal
  With head rotation and pressure on carotid sinus (as in tumors, shaving, and tight collars)
  After exertion

Syncope due to orthostatic hypotension
  After standing up
  Temporal relationship with start of medication leading to hypotension or changes of dosage
  Prolonged standing, especially in crowded and hot places
  Presence of autonomic neuropathy or Parkinsonism
  After exertion

Cardiac syncope
  Presence of definite structural heart disease
  During exertion or supine
  Preceded by palpitation
  Family history of sudden death

Cerebrovascular syncope
  With arm exercise
  Differences in blood pressure or pulse in the two arms

---

trying to get to the toilet. Profuse sweating, light-headedness, and myoclonic jerking are frequent. Some subjects reported nightmares immediately before the episode.

After regaining consciousness most subjects felt very weak and could not remain upright, but were oriented. The frequency of attacks varied from weekly to annually, and most subjects also had daytime episodes, which sounded vasovagal in nature. Sometimes, bradycardia was documented during nocturnal syncope. One subject, who was fortuitously monitored during a spontaneous nocturnal episode, had electrocardiographic (ECG) and encephalographic (EEG) findings that were consistent with vasovagal syncope. Tilt-table testing without drug provocation has been positive in about 60% of the subjects. There is no tongue biting, postictal confusion, automatism, or dystonic posturing. Nevertheless, it is most important to differentiate nocturnal syncope from atypical forms of epilepsy, such as abdominal epilepsy or other types of complex partial seizure disorder.

How are we to confirm the diagnosis? Clearly, simultaneous ECG, EEG, and blood pressure recordings during nocturnal episodes would be pivotal. However, these nocturnal episodes are difficult to capture because they are typically very brief and unpredictable. In most cases, a detailed patient history, and the exclusion of other possibilities, may be the most reliable and practicable way of making the diagnosis. However, a neurological consultation is mandatory. If the clinical picture is not typical, cardiac syncope should be considered.

In terms of frequency, nocturnal syncope may be more frequent than is currently supposed (based on the literature) since establishing the diagnosis is so difficult. Potentially, implantable monitors may open the door to successful assessment of greater numbers of affected individuals.

Syncope in older subjects

In the 2004 Guidelines, it is reported that in older patients the common prodromes or warning symptoms suggestive of vasovagal syncope are less frequent than in younger individuals. Consequently, laboratory autonomic assessment (i.e., carotid sinus massage and tilt-table testing) become more relevant for establishing the diagnosis, even if indirect [1]. The results of a recent Italian multicenter study provide support for this statement [4].

A total of 485 consecutive patients with unexplained syncope were divided into two predefined age groups: 224 patients <65 years and 261 patients ≥65 years. The clinical features of syncope were analyzed using a standard 46-item data form. The diagnosis of the cause of syncope was possible on the basis of history alone in 26% of younger patients but only 5% older ones ($p < 0.0001$). Younger patients had a longer duration of prodromal symptoms. The frequency of prodromal symptoms (especially autonomic ones, such as a diaphoresis, nausea, and feeling of cold) was significantly higher in the younger patients than in the older ones. Furthermore, in the younger group, the frequency of palpitations was higher than that observed in the older group. On the other hand, older patients more frequently experienced incontinence and trauma during loss of consciousness. Even during the recovery phase the frequency of autonomic symptoms was higher in younger patients. So, during the prodromal and recovery phases the frequency of symptoms was substantially less in older subjects. The dilemma then is that, in older patients, the clinical features of cardiac and neurally-mediated reflex syncope are very similar. This finding, together with the higher prevalence of heart disease in older individuals, undermines the utility of the medical history in differentiating between a cardiac and neurally-mediated cause of syncope in older patients.

Laughter-induced syncope

A laughter-induced fall has been mainly attributed to cataplexy, defined as a complete loss of muscular control triggered by emotions (usually laughter). Even when the patient appears to be wholly unconscious, there is full recollection of all events later. Cataplexy most often occurs as part of narcolepsy; in fact, the combination of cataplexy with daytime sleepiness ensures the diagnosis of narcolepsy.

Laughing is not typically considered a trigger for neurally-mediated reflex syncope. However, some cases of laughter-induced syncope have been reported recently [5–8]. The age of the patients ranged from 12 to 63 years. One healthy subject reported by Sarzi Braga and Pedretti [6] had a 20-year history of syncope preceded by intense laughter. During tilt-table testing a mixed vasovagal response (i.e., combined cardioinhibitory and vasodepressor) was induced and the patient recognized the typical prodromal symptoms. In another case, a girl with Angelman syndrome had recurrent episodes of loss of consciousness associated with asystole (up to 11 s) after outbursts of laughing during which there may have been obstructed expiration, probably caused by contraction of the laryngeal muscles [7]. This results in a Valsalva-like maneuver that may trigger the vagal reaction.

The mechanism of laughter-induced syncope is unknown. However, during the Valsalva-like maneuver a sudden drop in blood pressure, in the absence of compensatory tachycardia, has been recorded. Perhaps, this mimics the laughter response in some individuals.

Laughter-related syncope is uncommon but, like supine syncope, it may be more frequent than what appears in the literature because it could be readily misdiagnosed as cataplexy. Sleep disorders must be excluded and a neurologic consultation is often mandatory.

Conclusion

The medical history remains the foundation of differentiating syncope from other forms of TLOC. In many cases the history is sufficient to provide the diagnosis; however, care must be taken. The circumstances of the clinical symptoms, along with the age of and associated morbidities in the patient, must be factored in by an experienced clinician before a final diagnosis is established.

References

1 Brignole M, Alboni P, Benditt DG, *et al.* Guidelines on management (diagnosis and treatment) of syncope—update 2004. *Europace* 2004;**6**:467–537.

2 Krediet CTP, Jardine DL, Cortelli P, Visman AGR, Wieling W. Vasovagal syncope interrupting sleep? *Heart* 2004;**90**:e25.

3 Jardine DL, Krediet CTP, Cortelli P, Wieling W. Fainting in your sleep? *Clin Auton Res* 2006;**16**:76–8.

4 Del Rosso A, Alboni P, Brignole M, Menozzi C, Raviele A. Relation of clinical presentation of syncope to the age of patients. *Am J Cardiol* 2005;**96**:1431–5.

5 Bloomfield D, Jazrawi S. Shear hilarity leading to laugh syncope in a healthy man. *JAMA* 2005;**293**:2863–4.
6 Sarzi Braga S, Pedretti RFE. Laugher-induced syncope. *Lancet* 2005;**366**:426.
7 Vanagt WY, Pulles-Heintzberger CF, Vernooy K, Cornelussen RN, Delhaas T. Asystole during outburst of laughing in a child with Angelman syndrome. *Pediatr Cardiol* 2005;**26**:866–8.
8 Bragg MJ. Fall about laughing: a case of laughter syncope. *Emerg Med Australas* 2006;**18**:518–19.

CHAPTER 7

Emergency department evaluation of transient loss of consciousness/syncope

François P Sarasin

Scope of the problem

Initial assessment of suspected transient loss of consciousness (including presumed syncope), frequently in emergency departments (EDs) settings, should include a careful clinical history and physical examination, supine and upright blood pressure measurements, and 12-lead electrocardiography (ECG) [1]. The diagnostic yield of this noninvasive evaluation ranges from 30 to 60%.

After ED assessment, indication for hospitalization is dictated by two objectives: diagnosis and therapy. If the cause of syncope is identified, hospitalization should depend on the underlying etiology and its specific risk, and the therapeutic purposes. While patients with cardiac syncope (arrhythmia, valvular disease, and here including pulmonary embolism) should be admitted, those with reflex or orthostatic syncope usually do not need admission, except in the presence of severe comorbidities. On the other hand, when evaluation does not reveal a clear etiology, physicians must determine which patients require diagnostic testing and in what setting it should occur. The fear of life-threatening complications, mainly arrhythmias, often prompts physicians to adopt a "safe" approach (i.e., minimize risk to the patient). Although hospitalization has low diagnostic yield and therapeutic benefits, this results in high admission rates and generates enormous health care costs [2].

Risk stratification research and limitations

Several studies have attempted to develop risk stratification tools for patients who present to the ED with an apparent syncope. Three studies derived and validated risk classification systems, predicting the risk of death and/or arrhythmias [3–5]. Markers found by all authors to predict adverse outcomes included (1) an abnormal ECG, (2) a history of congestive heart failure (CHF),

Syncope and Transient Loss of Consciousness, 1st edition. Edited by David G Benditt *et al.*
© 2007 Blackwell Publishing, ISBN: 978-1-4051-7625-5.

and (3) age greater than 45 or 65 years. In single studies, the absence of pro-drome before syncope and a history of ventricular arrhythmias also predicted the 1-year risk of death and arrhythmias. Patients with none of these risk factors had death and/or arrhythmia event rates ranging between 0 and 7%.

The most important limitation of these studies, however, was an inappropriate time frame for assessing adverse events. Prediction instruments for long-term outcomes may not be helpful for ED decision making, since emergency physicians are concerned about the occurrence of short-term events requiring immediate hospitalizations. Other limitations include selection biases, variations in follow-up methods, and absence of quantifying how these instruments change clinical practice.

Quinn *et al.* derived and validated a decision rule predicting the 7-day risk of serious outcomes [6]. Predictors included an abnormal ECG, complaint of shortness of breath, hematocrit $\leq 30\%$, systolic blood pressure ≤ 90 mmHg, and a history of CHF. This rule was 98% sensitive (95% CI 89–100) and 56% specific (95% CI 52–60) to predict the short-term risks of death, myocardial infarction, arrhythmias, pulmonary embolism, stroke, subarachnoid hemor-rhage, and internal bleeding, and return ED visit. This study, however, has limitations. First, the population included both syncope and near-syncope patients. Near syncope can encompass different symptoms, such as weakness or dizziness, which may limit the generalizability of the observations. Second, the selected outcomes included conditions, such as subarachnoid hemorrhage, gastrointestinal bleeding, or sepsis. Predicting those events, usually obvious after initial evaluation, has limited clinical value. Finally, the rule did not include age as a predictor, although studies suggest that age is strongly asso-ciated with adverse events.

Shen *et al.* hypothesized that a designated "syncope unit" in the ED, equipped with diagnostic resources facilitating diagnostic assessment of com-mon causes of syncope (e.g., cardiac testing, tilt-table testing), would improve the diagnostic yield and reduce admission rate, compared with standard care [7]. Eligible patients included those generally considered for hospital admis-sion and presenting "intermediate-risk factors," such as an abnormal but non-diagnostic ECG, underlying heart disease, or a clinical history suggesting car-diac syncope. The results showed that (1) the diagnostic yield increased from 10 to 67%, (2) hospital admission was reduced from 98 to 43%, and (3) this strategy was safe. Transfer of this experience from a single tertiary-care center to community hospitals' EDs remains to be demonstrated.

Current recommendations

Position papers provide recommendations about the need for hospitalization [1, 8]. Admission for diagnostic purpose (i.e., the initial evaluation revealed no clear etiology) is recommended if stratification indicates that a patient is at risk for cardiac syncope. Factors that lead to stratification as high risk for serious outcomes include (1) underlying heart disease, (2) abnormal ECG, (3) family history of sudden death, (4) syncope occurring during exercise or caus-ing severe injury, and (5) any clinical features suggesting cardiac syncope. Of note, an age threshold was not suggested. Although retrospective, recent rec-ommendations suggest that compared with current practice, applying these criteria would lead to a significant reduction in hospitalizations rates [9].

Perspectives

The decision to hospitalize a patient with syncope for diagnostic evaluation depends mainly on the short-term risk of adverse events. However, major gaps exist in the knowledge of the epidemiology of these adverse events. Such data are critical for understanding the potential benefit offered by hospitalization. Studies aiming to quantify the occurrence of short-term adverse events rate and identifying risk factors for these events are clearly needed. Such data would provide the foundation for randomized trials demonstrating the effectiveness and safety of outpatient evaluation.

References

1 Brignole M, Alboni P, Benditt DG, et al.; Task Force on Syncope, European Society of Car-diology. Guidelines on management (diagnosis and treatment) of syncope. *Eur Heart J* 2004;**25**:2054–72.
2 Sun BC, Edmond JA, Camargo CA, Jr. Direct medical costs of syncope-related hospitaliza-tions in the United States. *Am J Cardiol* 2005;**95**:668–71.
3 Martin TP, Hanusa BH, Kapoor WN. Risk stratification of patients with syncope. *Ann Emerg Med* 1997;**29**:459–66.
4 Colavicchi F, Ammirati F, Melina D, et al. Development and prospective validation of a risk stratification system for patients with syncope in the emergency department: the OESIL risk score. *Eur Heart J* 2003;**24**:811–19.
5 Sarasin FP, Hanusa BH, Perneger TV, et al. A risk score to predict arrhythmias in patients with unexplained syncope. *Acad Emerg Med* 2003;**10**:1312–17.
6 Quinn J, McDermott D, Stiell I, et al. Prospective validation of the San Francisco syncope rule to predict patients with serious outcomes. *Ann Emerg Med* 2006;**47**:455–6.
7 Shen W, Decker W, Smars P, et al. Syncope evaluation in the emergency departments (SEEDS): a multidisciplinary approach to syncope management. *Circulation* 2004;**10**:3636–45.
8 Huff SJ, Decker WW, Quinn JV, et al., for the American College of Emergency Physicians Clinical Policies Subcommittee. Clinical policy: critical issues in the evaluation and man-agement of adult patients presenting with syncope. *Ann Emerg Med* 2007;**49**:431–44.
9 Elesber AA, Decker WW, Smars PA, et al. Impact of the application of the American College of Emergency Physicians recommendations for the admission of syncopal patients on a retrospectively studied population presenting to the emergency department. *Am Heart J* 2005;**149**:826–31.

CHAPTER 8

The essential autonomic assessment for evaluating the cause of syncope

Carlos A Morillo, Juan C Guzman

Acute or chronic alterations in autonomic regulation of heart rate and blood pressure play an important role in patients with recurrent syncope, particularly in those without evidence of significant cardiac abnormality. As a result, autonomic function tests are an important tool for the assessment of syncope [1].

The history and physical examination remains the cornerstone for the initial assessment of the patient with recurrent syncope. Autonomic disorders that may present with syncope include disorders with primary intermittent alterations in autonomic function, such as neurally-mediated reflex syncope (vasovagal faint and carotid sinus syndrome), and autonomic dysfunction causing chronic orthostatic intolerance or secondary intermittent alterations usually triggered by drugs or toxins [2]. Finally, diseases that result in progressive and permanent autonomic failure (diabetes, pure autonomic failure, multiple system atrophy, and systemic disease) should also be assessed with autonomic function tests to determine the level of the disturbance.

This chapter will review the current role of autonomic testing in patients with recurrent unexplained syncope.

Orthostatic stress

Assessing the response of blood pressure and heart rate to postural changes remains the simplest and most effective autonomic test. Both passive (standing) and active (head-up tilt) tests have been used to determine autonomic reflex response to orthostatic stress [3]:

1 *Standing test*: Evaluation of the response of blood pressure and heart rate immediately after assuming the upright position is a simple test that should be performed routinely in patients with syncope and the suspicion of orthostatic hypotension and other orthostatic intolerance syndromes, such as inappropriate sinus tachycardia (IST) and postural orthostatic tachycardia syndrome

Syncope and Transient Loss of Consciousness, 1st edition. Edited by David G Benditt *et al.*

(POTS). Blood pressure and heart rate should be recorded on a beat-to-beat basis to identify changes and at a minimum should be measured after 30 seconds and at 1 and 3 minutes after assuming the upright position. We recommend performing another measurement 5 minutes after assuming the upright position particularly in elderly patients due to the potential of delayed orthostatic hypotension [3]. Increased heart rate followed by a relative bradycardia, if present, is observed usually between 15 and 30 seconds after assuming the upright position. This response is mediated by both vagal withdrawal and increased sympathetic outflow to the sinus node and is assessed by estimating the $R - R_{max}/R - R_{min}$ ratio [4, 5]. Blood pressure should also be assessed preferably on a beat-to-beat basis. This test rarely leads to syncope. However, presyncope can be observed in patients with significant orthostatic hypotension.

Orthostatic hypotension is defined as a drop in systolic blood pressure >20 mmHg and/or in diastolic blood pressure >10 mmHg. Heart rate is usually unchanged or slightly increased in patients with neurogenic orthostatic hypotension associated or not with symptoms [6]. Other responses may include an increase in heart rate >30 bpm without changes in blood pressure. This response identifies patients with either POTS or IST (Figure 8.1).

2 *Head-up tilt test*: Head-up tilt test (HUT) was introduced in 1986 for the assessment of patients with syncope of unknown etiology [7]. HUT is useful to identify subjects with either vasovagal syncope or other orthostatic intolerance syndromes, including POTS, IST, and neurogenic forms of orthostatic hypotension, such as pure autonomic failure and multiple systemic atrophy.

There is no consensus on the ideal HUT protocol and this is the main limitation of this test. The European Society of Cardiology (ESC) Task Force on Syncope recommends a HUT protocol that includes a passive phase performed without the administration of provocative agents and that should last at least 20 minutes [8]. If the patient remains asymptomatic, a sublingual or spray dose of nitroglycerine (400 μg) or intravenous incremental isoproterenol infusion is administered during another 15 minutes or until syncope is induced. Several responses have been described, which include the following:

1 *Dysautonomic pattern* is characterized by a progressive reduction in blood pressure and pulse pressure without changes in heart rate that may progress to a syncopal response. This response is frequently observed in the elderly and is associated with acute and chronic pure autonomic failure, as well as multiple system atrophy.

2 *Postural orthostatic tachycardia* is associated with a rise in heart rate, usually accompanied by a sense of rapid heart beating by the patient, and with other symptoms of orthostatic intolerance.

3 *Vasovagal* response is characterized by sudden drop in blood pressure and heart rate. Typical response patterns in patients with vasovagal syncope have been characterized by the ESC and are defined by hemodynamic changes: systolic arterial pressure <70 mmHg and/or bradycardia associated with syncope that resembles the clinical presentation [8].

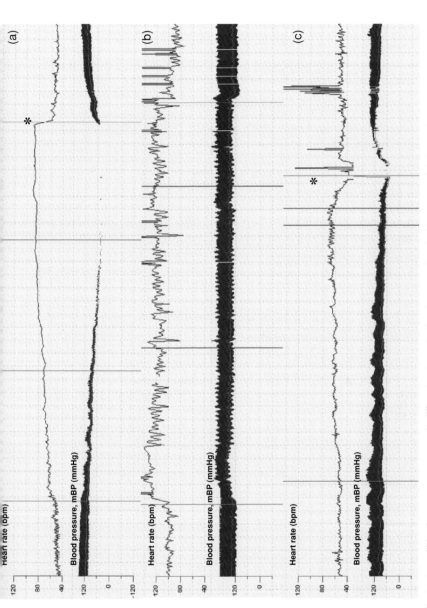

Figure 8.1 Heart rate and blood pressure responses in different autonomic disorders associated with syncope: (a) Beat-to-beat heart rate and blood pressure in an 85-year-old patient with typical dysautonomic response, and a sustained increase in heart rate from 50 to 80 bpm observed associated with a marked progressive reduction in blood pressure and marked reduction in pulse pressure up to the induction of syncope.* (b) Response in a 20-year-old female with chronic orthostatic intolerance. Heart rate >30 bpm (90–120 bpm) is triggered by tilting at 70° and is maintained at this level without changes in blood pressure throughout the duration of the study. This pattern is typical of POTS. (c) Vasovagal syncope* during tilt characterized by abrupt onset of bradycardia and hypotension typical of a mixed response.

Carotid sinus massage

Carotid sinus massage (CSM) is a simple test that is recommended for the assessment of unexplained syncope in patients over 40 years with unexplained syncope [7].

CSM should be performed in the supine and upright positions (usually on a tilt table) under continuous electrocardiographic and blood pressure monitoring [8]. CSM should be performed for 5–10 seconds at the anterior margin of the sternocleidomastoid muscle at the level of the cricoid cartilage. Massage of the opposite side should be performed after 1 or 2 minutes [8]. If an asystolic response is evoked, atropine (1 mg or 0.02 mg/kg) should be administered to evaluate the vasodepressor component. CSM should be repeated in the upright position if asystole is not triggered in the supine position [9]. As it carries potential hazards, CSM should be performed by experienced physicians who are aware of the potential complications [7].

A positive response is defined by the induction of a ventricular pause >3 seconds and/or a fall in systolic blood pressure >50 mmHg. The response to CSM may be either cardioinhibitory (i.e., asystole) or vasodepressor (fall in systolic blood pressure), or mixed. CSM should be avoided in patients with previous strokes or transient ischemic attacks within the past 3 months (except if carotid Doppler studies excluded significant stenosis) or patients with carotid bruits.

Catecholamine determinations

Catecholamine determinations in the supine and upright position are useful to determine the presence of either hyper- or hypoadrenergic states. Norepinephrine levels in the upright position are markedly elevated (>600 pg) in patients with POTS and less so in IST [3]. In patients with neurogenic orthostatic hypotension, norepinephrine levels are reduced both at rest and after orthostatic stress with markedly blunted response in patients with pure autonomic failure [10].

References

1 Mathias CJ, Deguchi K, Schatz I. Observations on recurrent syncope and presyncope in 641 patients. *Lancet* 2001;**357**:348–53.

2 Mathias CJ. Role of autonomic evaluation in the diagnosis and management of syncope. *Clin Auton Res* 2004;**14**:145–54.

3 Grubb BP, Vesga BE, Guzman JC, Silva FA, Morillo CA. Autonomic dysfunction syndromes associated with orthostatic intolerance. *Biomedical* 2003;**23**:103–14.

4 Wieling W, Borst C, van Brederode JF, *et al.* Testing for autonomic neuropathy: heart rate changes after orthostatic manoeuvres and static muscle contractions. *Clin Sci* 1983;**64**:581–6.

5 Wieling W, Borst C, van Lieshout JJ, *et al*. Assessment of methods to estimate impairment of vagal and sympathetic innervation of the heart in diabetic neuropathy. *Neth J Med* 1985;**28**:383–92.

6 Schatz IJ, Bannister RM, Freeman RL, *et al*. Consensus statement on the definition of orthostatic hypotension, pure autonomic failure and multiple systemic atrophy. *Clin Auton Res* 1996;**6**:125–6.

7 Kenny RA, Ingram A, Bayliss J, Sutton R. Head-up tilt: a useful test for investigating unexplained syncope. *Lancet* 1986;**1**:1352–5.

8 Brignole M, Alboni P, Benditt DG, *et al*. Guidelines on management (diagnosis and treatment) of syncope—update 2004. *Europace* 2004;**6**:467–537.

9 Morillo CA, Camacho ME, Word MA, Gilligan DM, Ellenbogen KA. Diagnostic utility of mechanical, pharmacological and orthostatic stimulation of the carotid sinus in patients with unexplained syncope. *J Am Coll Cardiol* 1999;**34**:1587–94.

10 Mabuchi N, Hirayama M, Koike Y, *et al*. Progression and prognosis in pure autonomic failure (PAF); comparison with multiple system atrophy. *J Neurol Neurosurg Psychiatry* 2005;**76**:947–52.

CHAPTER 9

Neurally-mediated reflex syncope: recognition by history and clinical testing*

Anna Serletis, Robert S Sheldon

The diagnosis of transient loss of consciousness poses interesting challenges. The etiologies most commonly considered include syncope and epileptic seizures, and the distinction between the two is not always accurately made. On the one hand, at least 40% of people will faint at least once in their lives [1]. On the other hand, approximately 3% of people will have one or more epileptic seizures in their lifetime [2]. Diagnostic tools aimed at differentiating between these causes of loss of consciousness, regardless of sensitivity and specificity, will struggle with either positive or negative predictive values because of this disproportionate distribution. Similarly, diagnostic challenges arise within different populations of people with syncope. In the community at large, but less so in clinic or hospital settings, vasovagal syncope is by far the most common diagnosis [3, 4]. It is generally benign and usually does not require specific treatment. Conversely, syncope secondary to causes such as cardiac arrhythmias, myocardial infarction, or heart block occasionally forebodes a fatal outcome that may be avoided with appropriate management [5].

The investigation of loss of consciousness can be costly and intrusive [5–8] and is often inconclusive or incorrect [3, 8–10]. Therefore, an early, accurate, efficient, and inexpensive method of diagnosing the etiology of such events is highly desirable.

Approach to syncope

The patient presenting with total loss of consciousness should be approached first with a thorough history and physical examination, accompanied by a

* This study was supported in part by grant 73-1976 from the Canadian Institute for Health Research, Ottawa, Ontario, Canada.

resting electrocardiogram. These two steps will provide an accurate diagnosis in the majority of cases without recourse to further testing. Only then should physicians consider more intensive investigation. Of the available tests two have a reasonable diagnostic yield: tilt-table testing and implantable loop recorders (ILRs).

Quantitative histories

The history remains the essential component of the investigation of loss of consciousness. Although other possibilities such as narcolepsy and cataplexy should be remembered, the initial diagnostic step usually is to determine whether the patient has syncope or epileptic seizures. Traditionally, characteristics such as auras, tongue biting, convulsive activity, and physical trauma are used to diagnose a seizure disorder; however, this can be misleading in patients with akinetic seizures or convulsive syncope. Zaidi *et al.* emphasized this dilemma, showing that approximately 26% of patients originally diagnosed with epilepsy were ultimately found to have vasovagal syncope as the cause of their loss of consciousness [10]. The diagnosis of syndromes of loss of consciousness has been particularly troublesome because the principal symptom is unconsciousness, and bystander histories are often not available. This frequently leads to detailed and often invasive investigations of patients with loss of consciousness.

Another difficulty may be the lack of structured, evidence-based histories. Physicians learn how to take histories from accumulation of anecdotes, from formal teaching (which occasionally lacks an evidential background), and from personal experience. However, nearly 20 years ago Van Donselaar's group reported that a structured history significantly improved the accuracy of the diagnosis of a first seizure. Histories should be based on quantitative evidence to be maximally credible. Several groups have contributed such evidence.

Calkins *et al.* studied a mixed population of 80 syncope patients with ventricular tachycardia, complete heart block, or vasovagal syncope to identify features within the clinical history that predicted the causes of syncope [11]. Each participant completed a standard questionnaire and a written description of the syncopal events. Four factors (age, sex, duration of the recovery period, and the presence of mild or severe fatigue after syncope) identified the cause of syncope with 98% sensitivity and 100% specificity.

Alboni *et al.* administered standard questionnaires to 341 patients with established causes of syncope to elicit historical data surrounding their syncopal events [4]. Among patients with known or suspected heart disease, the most specific features of cardiac syncope were loss of consciousness while supine or during effort, blurred vision, and convulsive syncope. The most important historical features of neurally-mediated syncope were time between the first and last episode >4 years, abdominal discomfort before loss of consciousness, and nausea and diaphoresis during recovery. Independently, heart disease predicted a cardiac cause of syncope with 95% sensitivity and 45% specificity. In patients without known heart disease, the only significant historical feature to suggest a cardiac etiology was palpitations before syncope.

These earlier studies illustrated the importance of historical features in classifying etiology of loss of consciousness. However, the results were reported as odds or risk ratios, which are not easy to use clinically. Furthermore, the populations were not divided into the three common problem areas: syncope versus seizures, syncope with structurally normal hearts, and syncope with structural heart disease. Accordingly, diagnostic point scores have been and are being developed to address these specific questions.

Calgary Syncope Symptom Study

The Calgary Syncope Symptom Study is a multinational, multicenter study that is developing standardized, evidence-based diagnostic questionnaires. These can be used in three specific situations. First, can vasovagal syncope be accurately distinguished from epilepsy? Second, in patients without known structural heart disease, can vasovagal syncope be distinguished from other causes of syncope? Finally, can accurate differentiation of vasovagal syncope and ventricular tachycardia be achieved in patients with known structural cardiac disease? A comprehensive questionnaire was administered to 671 patients in three academic centers in Canada and Wales, and point scores were developed with logistic regression analysis.

The first criteria to be developed were to distinguish between syncope and seizures [12]. The cause of loss of consciousness was known in 539 patients (according to gold-standard criteria), and it included various types of epilepsy, vasovagal syncope, and cardiac arrhythmias. A point score to differentiate syncope from seizures was derived, which proved to have a sensitivity of 94% and a specificity of 94%.

Significant historical aspects suggestive of seizure activity included preceding emotional stress, "déjà vu" or "jamais vu," head turning or unusual posturing or motor activity during an event, confusion upon awakening, or tongue laceration. Conversely, syncope was favored by the presence of the following features: separate episodes of presyncope, preceding diaphoresis, or event precipitated by prolonged standing or sitting. The point score was independent of the number of losses of consciousness and length of history, suggesting that it could be used quite early in the patient's clinical course. It also correctly identified most patients with syncope of unknown origin. Interestingly, the point score functions in the same fashion as a skilled clinician, weighing the evidence both for and against competing diagnostic possibilities.

The second point score focused on syncope and no known structural disease—a very common clinical problem [13]. The gold-standard populations had proven causes of syncope. The accuracy of the decision rule was assessed with bootstrapping, and data sets were complete for all subjects. The causes of syncope were known in 323 patients, and these included tilt-positive vasovagal syncope (235 patients) and other diagnoses such as complete heart block and supraventricular tachycardias (88 patients). The point score correctly classified 90% of patients, diagnosing vasovagal syncope with 89% sensitivity and 91% specificity. Features against vasovagal syncope included a history of bifascicular block or complete heart block, supraventricular tachycardia, diabetes, observed cyanosis during syncope, and having a first syncopal spell after the age of 35 years. Indeed, this single criterion is very accurate for distinguishing between vasovagal syncope and other causes [14]. Factors in favor of vasovagal syncope included presyncope or syncope with orthostatic stress, pain, or medical settings, and a prodrome of warmth or diaphoresis. Once again, the point score functions like a skilled clinician, weighing the evidence for and against competing diagnostic possibilities. Later, use of the point score suggested that 68% of patients with syncope of unknown cause and a negative tilt-table test have vasovagal syncope. Preliminary results from a Columbian study have confirmed its accuracy in a population that differs both culturally and linguistically.

The questionnaire is simple and easy to use, taking less than 1 minute to complete. With it, the use of tilt-table tests in the Calgary Syncope Clinic has dropped by over 90%, and they are now used mainly for difficult diagnostic challenges characterized by the need to know hemodynamic changes during orthostatic stress or electroencephalogram changes during unconsciousness. The questionnaire's ease of use was demonstrated in a recent study of the effect of family history on the likelihood of having vasovagal syncope [1]. The questionnaire was administered by a medical student in spare time to 112 medical students and first-degree relatives in a 10-week span, allowing information to be accurately and efficiently collected about historical features of the syncopal events of entire families, despite geographic separation. To complete 112 tilt-table tests would have taken a somewhat longer period with more resources. The use of the questionnaire in this study emphasized the value of a point score in clinical research and yielded important results regarding the role of family history and gender in one's likelihood of experiencing vasovagal syncope.

Similarly, the Prevention of Syncope Trial II (POST II) uses the Calgary Syncope Symptom Score as an entry criterion [15]. This multicenter, international, randomized control trial is testing the effectiveness of fludrocortisone in the prevention of vasovagal syncope. The symptom score was chosen rather than tilt-table tests as an inclusion criterion, due to the accessibility of this diagnostic tool to emergency physicians and community physicians, the objective and accurate diagnostic criteria, and its rapidity of administration. The intent is to move the diagnosis and treatment of syncope out of the offices of specialists and into general medical clinics.

Eventually, use of these and similar diagnostic criteria should increase the intersite reliability and feasibility of large multicenter studies, by providing standardized patient eligibility. However there are questions yet to be asked. Does this work as well in older patients as in younger ones? This is important because most European studies report syncope populations with mean ages around 60 years, while North American syncope populations have reported ages 15–20 years younger. How well do the scores perform in emergency wards? Do we need to derive specific scores for patients with genetic arrhythmias? And are these scores accurate across cultural and linguistic divides?

Syncope risk stratification

There are times, particularly in the emergency room, when it is more efficient and timely to simply know the prognosis of the patient rather than the precise diagnosis. This facilitates safe decisions about admission to hospital or discharge from the emergency ward. The role of standard questionnaires for patients presenting with loss of consciousness not only facilitates diagnosis, but also synthesizes important prognostic information and aid with risk stratification. Kapoor's group studied 497 patients in a variety of ambulatory and acute care settings, following them for up to a year [16]. Although electrocardiographic abnormalities and the absence of prodromal nausea and vomiting predicted arrhythmic syncope, only the presence of structural heart disease predicted death.

The OESIL1 study, performed by Colivicchi *et al.*, also developed criteria that could predict life-threatening causes of syncope in patients presenting to the emergency room [9]. A cohort of 270 patients was used to derive the following predictors of mortality: age over 65 years, a history of cardiovascular disease, syncope without prodromes, and an abnormal ECG. The number of predictors present was found to predict a staggering range of mortality risk, from 0 to 57% in 1 year. This scoring system was subsequently tested and validated in a cohort of 328 patients, yielding very similar mortality patterns. Of course this score may not require syncope at all; it may simply be a general rule for overall medical risk. It awaits successful confirmation in other geographic areas.

The San Francisco Syncope Rule [17] similarly aimed to identify patients presenting with syncope who are at risk for serious short-term outcomes. With 98% sensitivity and 56% specificity, the following factors were predictive of short-term serious outcomes: history of congestive heart failure, hematocrit <30%, abnormal ECG, shortness of breath, and an initial systolic blood pressure <90 mmHg. It was subsequently confirmed in a second population. Again, these may simply be factors of overall high medical risk and have little to do with syncope. At least four of the factors are common in high-risk cardiovascular patients.

Tilt-table tests and implantable loop recorders

After ECGs the two tests most favored for the investigation of syncope are tilt-table tests and ILRs. Both have contributed invaluable insights into the physiology and clinical course of patients with syncope of uncertain origin. Tilt-table tests have been the foundation for syncope studies in the last 25 years. However, although they seem simple, they do contain numerous variables that affect study outcome [18]. These include the angle and duration of head-up tilt, the type and dose of drug challenge, the number of head-up phases during the test, and subject hydration and age. The tests do not always faithfully reproduce the subject's clinical symptoms, and the hemodynamic criteria vary widely and are rarely based on evidence. Critically, tilt-table tests have not been validated against "gold-standard" populations, and different tilt-table test protocols identify patient populations that do not overlap completely. Which test is true? Can we diagnose patients with a test that appears to diagnose only a subset of truly positive patients? These many factors suggest that the future of tilt-table testing lies in physiologic studies and in patients with diagnoses that are refractory to a good history.

ILRs may play a similar role. They have been invaluable in establishing the outcomes of patients at elevated risk for arrhythmic syncope and have provided variable information about the heart rate of patients with probable vasovagal syncope during their spells [7]. However the predominant rhythm during vasovagal syncope, epileptic seizures, pseudosyncope, and pseudoseizures is sinus rhythm, and therefore the main use of loop recorders in the diagnosis of syndromes of loss of consciousness may be in patients with diagnoses that are refractory to a good history and in whom an arrhythmic cause should be considered. The ILR also has potential problems. It is a passive tool that relies on the patient having another syncopal spell. While this may be tolerable to many patients, it is not likely to be useful in patients with potentially fatal causes of syncope, and therefore its use may be practically restricted to patients deemed to be more likely than not to have a benign cause of syncope. Therefore, the loop recorder is unlikely to find a niche in diagnosing patients with dangerous causes of syncope and may simply detect sinus rhythm in many patients with vasovagal syncope. Whether it can be used to select patients for specific treatments of vasovagal syncope remains to be determined.

Future priorities

The adoption of quantitative histories and point score systems requires several more steps. First, do these point scores perform well in the very young and in the aged? Although this has not been systematically addressed, Ungar *et al.* concluded that the European Society of Cardiology guidelines on syncope can be accurately applied to elderly patients, even beyond the age of 90 years [19].

Second, do we need to derive specific scores for patients with genetic arrhythmias? Although these are usually detected after sustained ventricular arrhythmias or with family histories, many of these patients will also have vasovagal syncope. Third, how well do the scores perform in emergency wards, or across cultural and linguistic divides? Finally, they will need to be tested in randomized trials compared with conventional investigations.

References

1 Serletis A, Rose S, Sheldon AG, Sheldon RS. Vasovagal syncope in medical students and their first-degree relatives. *Eur Heart J* 2006;**27**(16):1965–70.

2 Chang BS, Lowenstein DH. Epilepsy. *N Engl J Med* 2003;**349**(13):1257–66.

3 Ammirati F, Colivicchi F, Santini M. Implementation of a simplified diagnostic algorithm in a multicentre prospective trial—the OESIL 2 Study (Osservatorio Epidemiologico della Sincope nel Lazio). *Eur Heart J* 2000;**21**:935–40.

4 Alboni P, Brignole M, Menozzi C, *et al*. Diagnostic value of history in patients with syncope with or without heart disease. *JACC* 2001;**37**(7):1921–8.

5 Brignole M, Alboni P, Benditt DG, *et al*. Task force report: guidelines on management (diagnosis and treatment) of syncope. *Eur Heart J* 2001;**22**(15):1256–306.

6 Pires LA, Ganji JR, Jarandila R, Steele R. Diagnostic patterns and temporal trends in the evaluation of adult patients hospitalized with syncope. *Arch Intern Med* 2001;**161**:1889–95.

7 Farwell DJ, Sulke AN. Does the use of a syncope diagnostic protocol improve the investigation and management of syncope? *Heart* 2004;**90**:52–8.

8 Shen WK, Decker WW, Smars PA, *et al*. Syncope Evaluation in the Emergency Department Study (SEEDS): a mulitdisciplinary approach to syncope management. *Circulation* 2004;**110**:3636–45.

9 Colivicchi F, Ammirati F, Melina D, *et al*. Development and prospective validation of a risk stratification system for patients with syncope in the emergency department: the OESIL risk score. *Eur Heart J* 2003;**24**:811–19.

10 Zaidi A, Clough P, Cooper P, *et al*. Misdiagnosis of epilepsy: many seizure-like attacks have a cardiovascular cause. *J Am Coll Cardiol* 2000;**36**:181–4.

11 Calkins H, Shyr Y, Frumin H, Schork A, Morady F. The value of the clinical history in the differentiation of syncope due to ventricular tachycardia, atrioventricular block, and neurocardiogenic syncope. *Am J Med* 1995;**98**:365–73.

12 Sheldon RS, Rose S, Ritchie D, *et al*. Historical criteria that distinguish syncope from seizures. *J Am Coll Cardiol* 2002;**40**(1):142–8.

13 Sheldon R, Rose S, Connolly S, *et al*. Diagnostic criteria for vasovagal syncope based on a quantitative history. *Eur Heart J* 2006;**27**:344–50.

14 Sheldon RS, Sheldon AG, Connolly SJ, *et al*. Age of first faint in patients with vasovagal syncope. *J Cardiovasc Electrophysiol* 2006;**17**(1):49–54.

15 Raj SR, Rose S, Ritchie D, Sheldon RS. The Second Prevention of Syncope Trial (POST II)—a randomized clinical trial of fludrocortisone for the prevention of neurally mediated syncope: rationale and study design. *Am Heart J* 2006;**151**:1186.e11–17.

16 Oh JH, Hanusa BH, Kapoor W. Do symptoms predict cardiac arrhythmias and mortality in patients with syncope? *Arch Intern Med* 1999;**159**:375–80.

17 Quinn JV, Stiell IG, McDermott DA, *et al*. Derivation of the San Franscico syncope rule to predict patients with short-term serious outcomes. *Ann Emerg Med* 2004;**43**:224–32.

18 Sheldon RS. Tilt testing for syncope: a reappraisal. *Curr Opin Cardiol* 2005;**20**(1):38–41.

19 Ungar A, Mussi C, Del Rosso A, *et al*. Diagnosis and characteristics of syncope in older patients referred to geriatric departments. *J Am Geriatr Soc* 2006;**54**:1531–6.

CHAPTER 10

Value and limitations of ambulatory electrocardiographic monitoring

Andrew D Krahn

Introduction

Cardiac monitoring is an essential diagnostic adjunct after the most important "test" in patients with syncope, a thorough history and physical examination [1]. Choice of investigative modalities is determined by the initial clinical evaluation, the frequency of symptoms, and the patient's ability to interact with the available monitoring technology [2]. Evolving technologies have provided a wide array of monitoring options for patients suspected of having cardiac arrhythmias, with each modality differing in duration of monitoring, quality of recording, convenience, and invasiveness.

Holter monitoring

Short-term electrocardiographic monitoring via 3–12-surface electrodes is the most common initial investigation in patients who present with syncope. Typically, this occurs in the emergency room or primary care setting with telemetry and continuous monitoring. The overall diagnostic yield of Holter monitoring is low: 4% in 2612 patients with symptoms of syncope or presyncope in a pooled analysis by Linzer *et al.* [3]. The major limiting factor in diagnosis of the index event is the likelihood of another syncopal episode during the monitoring period. Holter monitoring can also be used as a strategy to exclude a significant arrhythmic cause of symptoms in the primary care setting. Presyncope is a more common event during ambulatory monitoring but is less likely to be associated with an arrhythmia [4].

The apparent diagnostic yield, albeit modest, of Holter monitoring presumably reflects relatively common use of the device in the primary care setting in patients with frequent symptoms; this scenario would be expected to facilitate a symptom–rhythm correlation, even though the recording duration is quite limited. This leads to selection bias in the referral population, as referred patients

Syncope and Transient Loss of Consciousness, 1st edition. Edited by David G Benditt *et al.*
© 2007 Blackwell Publishing, ISBN: 978-1-4051-7625-5.

tend to have failed short-term monitoring, suggesting infrequent symptoms and the need for long-term monitoring strategies.

External loop recorders

An external cardiac loop recorder continuously records and stores an external single modified limb-lead electrogram with a 4–18-minute memory buffer. After the onset of spontaneous symptoms, the patient activates the device, which stores the previous 3–14 minutes, and the following 1–4 minutes, of recorded information. The captured rhythm strip can subsequently be uploaded and analyzed, and it often provides critical information regarding the onset of the arrhythmia. This system can be used for weeks to months, provided weekly battery changes are performed. The recording device is attached with two leads to the patient's chest wall and needs to be removed for bathing or showering, and it can be uncomfortable during sleep. A randomized trial has shown cost-effective diagnostic superiority to Holter monitors (22% for Holter monitoring vs 56% for the loop recorder, $p < 0.01$) [5]. A recent report suggests an increment in diagnostic yield when automatic activation is added to patient activation [6]. Similarly, a continuous monitor that transmits to a central monitoring station staffed by health professionals (so-called mobile cardiac outpatient telemetry), including full-time electrocardiographic monitor technicians, has recently come to the fore in the United States (Cardionet, San Diego, CA) and has shown incremental benefit to a standard external loop recorder in diagnosing or excluding arrhythmia [7].

Long-term compliance with external recording devices can be challenging because of electrode and skin-related problems and waning of patient motivation in the absence of recurrent symptoms. Nonetheless, some form of external monitoring is warranted in most patients because of the noninvasive and cost-effective nature of external recording devices.

Implantable loop recorders

The implantable loop recorder (ILR) permits prolonged monitoring without external electrodes. It is ideally suited to patients with infrequent recurrent syncope thought to be due to an arrhythmic cause. Similar to the external loop recorder, it is designed to correlate physiology with recorded cardiac rhythms, but it is implanted and therefore devoid of surface electrodes and accompanying compliance issues. The current ILR (Medtronic Reveal Plus® Model 9526) has a battery life of 18–24 months. The device is implanted subcutaneously in the chest wall under local anesthetic with antibiotic prophylaxis. The ILR has programmable automatic detection of rapid and slow heart rate episodes as well as pauses. A classification system for recorded events has been proposed by Brignole *et al.* [8] that categorizes the probable mechanism of syncope according to the pattern of bradycardia recorded during spontaneous episodes. This classification is useful for research purposes for event classification and is likely to prove useful in directing therapy once validated.

Currently, there are several studies establishing the utility of ILR in the diagnosis of syncope, including two randomized trials suggesting that the ILR is superior to conventional testing in patients with unexplained syncope and preserved left ventricular function [9, 10]. A recent prospective, multicenter observational study (International Study on Syncope of Uncertain Etiology 2, ISSUE-2) investigated the efficacy of therapies based on ILR diagnosis of recurrent suspected neurocardiogenic syncope [11]. Patients were included in the study if they experienced three or more clinically severe syncopal episodes over 2 years without significant electrocardiographic or cardiac abnormalities and presumably had vasovagal syncope. The 1-year recurrence rate among the 53 patients assigned to an ILR-specific therapy was 10% compared with 41% in the patients without specific therapy. The authors concluded that a strategy based on diagnostic information from early ILR implant, with therapy delayed until documentation of syncope, allows safe, specific, and effective therapy in patients with neurocardiogenic syncope. This trial has given "birth" to the ISSUE-3 study, which will randomize the pacing portion of the same format of study to assess an ILR-selected pacing response objectively.

Strategies for choosing prolonged monitoring

The literature clearly supports the use of the ILR in patients with recurrent unexplained syncope, who have failed a noninvasive workup and continue to have episodes. This represents a select group that has been referred for further testing, where ongoing symptoms are likely and a symptom–rhythm correlation is a feasible goal. The optimal patient for prolonged monitoring with an external or implantable loop recorder has symptoms suspicious of arrhythmia. ISSUE-2 suggests that documentation of the cardioinhibitory component of vasovagal syncope may identify a group of patients that respond well to pacing. After clinical assessment including determination of left ventricular function, a decision must be made if the underlying condition may represent a ventricular arrhythmia warranting consideration of an implantable cardioverter-defibrillator (Figure 10.1). All reports using the ILR have suggested a low incidence of life-threatening arrhythmia or significant morbidity with a prolonged monitoring strategy. This suggests a good prognosis for patients with recurrent unexplained syncope in the absence of left ventricular dysfunction or with negative electrophysiologic testing. Lastly, syncope fails to recur during long-term monitoring in almost one-third of patients even in the presence of frequent episodes prior to loop recorder implantation. This suggests that the cause of syncope in some instances is self-limited, reflecting a transient physiologic abnormality.

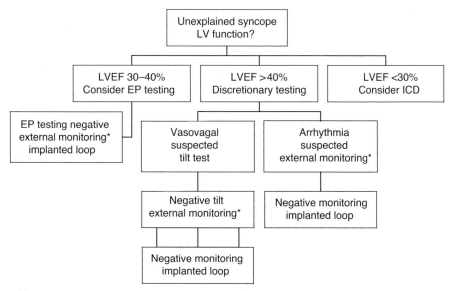

Figure 10.1 Approach to the use of cardiac monitoring in patients with unexplained syncope. Note that the presence and severity of left ventricular disease is assessed early to establish risk of sudden death and triage further investigation. EP, electrophysiology. The term 'external monitoring' (*) refers to long-term ECG monitoring such as 30-day event recorders or Mobile Cardiac Outpatient Telemetry (Cardionet Inc, San Diego, California). Short-term monitors (e.g., Holter monitoring) is not usually effective.

Conclusion

The ultimate diagnostic goal is to correlate symptoms to rhythm disturbances, and accurate attainment of this goal requires the judicious use of monitoring strategies. Ambulatory cardiac monitoring has provided a powerful means to elucidate etiology of presyncope or syncope. The choice of ambulatory monitoring strategies is governed by index of suspicion of cardiac arrhythmias, frequency and nature of symptoms, and accuracy of the monitoring device.

References

1 Sheldon R, Rose S, Ritchie D, *et al*. Historical criteria that distinguish syncope from seizures. *J Am Coll Cardiol* 2002;**40**(1):142–8.

2 Gula LJ, Krahn AD, Massel D, Skanes A, Yee R, Klein GJ. External loop recorders: determinants of diagnostic yield in patients with syncope. *Am Heart J* 2004;**147**(4):644–8.

3 Linzer M, Yang EH, Estes NA, Wang P, Vorperian VR, Kapoor WN. Diagnosing syncope. Part 2: Unexplained syncope. Clinical Efficacy Assessment Project of the American College of Physicians [see comments]. *Ann Intern Med* 1997;**127**:76–86.

4 Krahn AD, Klein GJ, Yee R, Skanes AC. Predictive value of presyncope in patients monitored for assessment of syncope. *Am Heart J* 2001;**141**:817–21.

5 Sivakumaran S, Krahn AD, Klein GJ, *et al*. A prospective randomized comparison of loop recorders versus Holter monitors in patients with syncope or presyncope. *Am J Med* 2003;**115**(1):1–5.

6 Reiffel JA, Schwarzberg R, Murry M. Comparison of autotriggered memory loop recorders versus standard loop recorders versus 24-hour Holter monitors for arrhythmia detection. *Am J Cardiol* 2005;**95**(9):1055–9.

7 Rothman SA, Laughlin JC, Seltzer J, *et al*. The diagnosis of cardiac arrhythmias: a prospective multi-center randomized study comparing mobile cardiac outpatient telemetry versus standard loop event monitoring. *J Cardiovasc Electrophysiol* 2007;**18**(3):241–7.

8 Brignole M, Moya A, Menozzi C, Garcia-Civera R, Sutton R. Proposed electrocardiographic classification of spontaneous syncope documented by an implantable loop recorder. *Europace* 2005;**7**(1):14–8.

9 Krahn AD, Klein GJ, Yee R, Hoch JS, Skanes AC. Cost implications of testing strategy in patients with syncope: randomized assessment of syncope trial. *J Am Coll Cardiol* 2003;**42**:495–501.

10 Farwell DJ, Sulke AN. Does the use of a syncope diagnostic protocol improve the investigation and management of syncope? *Heart* 2004;**90**(1):52–8.

11 Brignole M, Sutton R, Menozzi C, *et al*. Early application of an implantable loop recorder allows effective specific therapy in patients with recurrent suspected neurally mediated syncope. *Eur Heart J* 2006;**27**(9):1085–92.

CHAPTER 11

Recording ambulatory blood pressure in the syncope and TLOC evaluation

Dietrich Andresen

The decrease in overall cerebral perfusion during syncope is usually caused by a decrease in systemic blood pressure. It follows then that blood pressure recording is of fundamental importance in the evaluation of spontaneous transient loss of consciousness (TLOC) episodes to determine whether in fact the patient is experiencing "syncope."

Blood pressure measurements are taken as single measurements at rest or under stress conditions. They are also used in the evaluation of provocation tests (orthostatic blood pressure measurement and head-up tilt-testing [HUT]) or may be performed continuously as ambulatory blood pressure monitoring (ABPM). The current and possible future significance of blood pressure measurement is the subject of this chapter.

Orthostatic intolerance

Autonomic dysfunction (sometimes abbreviated as "dysautonomia") is the leading cause of orthostatic intolerance and may be severe enough to trigger cerebral hypoperfusion and loss of consciousness. The clinical syndromes of dysautonomia may be either acute or chronic. Although these have different mechanisms, they share the common feature of a drop in systemic blood pressure upon exposure to increased gravitational stress (e.g., standing up from seated or supine position).

What do we find in the guidelines [1]?
"The initial evaluation of a patient with syncope consists of a careful history and a physical examination, including orthostatic blood pressure measurements. Orthostatic syncope is diagnosed when there is documentation of orthostatic hypotension associated with syncope or presyncope." Unfortunately, the guideline document fails to mention that the diagnostic value

Syncope and Transient Loss of Consciousness, 1st edition. Edited by David G Benditt *et al.*
© 2007 Blackwell Publishing, ISBN: 978-1-4051-7625-5.

of the blood pressure measurement is restricted to those scenarios in which orthostatic syncope is suggested by the medical history. Only then is an abnormal test result specific for the presence of orthostatic syncope. An asymptomatic decrease in systolic blood pressure of >20 mmHg or an asymptomatic decrease in systolic blood pressure to <90 mmHg (defined as orthostatic hypotension) should not be taken as evidence for a cause of syncope if the medical history is inconsistent with such a diagnosis.

The nature of the orthostatic response to active standing is different from that of passive standing. Nonetheless, some authors perform only HUT (i.e., a passive standing test) on these patients. We primarily use the "active" standing test, as this presumably better reflects the mechanism of orthostatic dysregulation in normal clinical practice. In this regard, active standing on the one hand triggers muscle pump activity that would be expected to diminish postural hypotension, while on the other hand requires greater muscle blood flow (than would be expected with passive tilt) that may aggravate the drop in blood pressure.

Like most tests for the clarification of the basis for syncope, the standing test is a provocation maneuver, allowing conclusions about the possible mechanism of spontaneous syncope. It is nevertheless only an assumption that the individual patient's spontaneous syncope has the same mechanism as the syncope during the standing test.

Neurally-mediated syncope

Neurally-mediated mechanisms account for or contribute to 50–80% of all syncopal episodes. There are a wide variety of triggers that may lead to the hypotension and bradycardia associated with neurally-mediated syncope (NMS). Although the diagnosis of NMS is principally based on the medical history, HUT is helpful in confirming the possible diagnosis.

There are various positive response patterns seen during HUT. The classic "vasovagal reaction" is characterized by a sudden onset of hypotension, with or without coexisting bradycardia (although the heart rate is almost never appropriately tachycardic given the severity of hypotension [i.e., relative bradycardia]).

In the case of patients thought to be susceptible to NMS, apart from the electrocardiogram (ECG), it is also very important to measure blood pressure continuously during HUT. The significance of HUT and the different blood pressure and heart rate reactions will be discussed in detail elsewhere (see Chapters 8 and 9). Like all provocative tests, HUT measures changes in physiological parameters under "unnatural conditions." Accordingly, one should be cautious with respect to transferring the HUT observations to the patient's normal clinical conditions. In particular, only limited inferences about the mechanisms of spontaneous syncope may be drawn on the basis of the mechanisms of the NMS reaction during HUT. For example, although syncope in HUT is triggered by a primarily vasodepressive reaction, spontaneous syncope may nonetheless be mainly due to a cardioinhibitory reaction [2].

Ambulatory blood pressure monitoring

ABPM is a widely used method for the continuous measurement of blood pressure and for recording its circadian rhythm and intraindividual spontaneous variability. The value of this method in the diagnosis and therapeutic control of patients with arterial hypertension is widely accepted [3]. There is also firm evidence that ABPM is a sensitive predictor of cardiovascular outcome. However, the diagnostic yield of ABPM in the clarification of syncope is poor. One reason for this is that blood pressure is recorded only at the relatively long intervals of 15–30 minutes, so that short-term fluctuations, as occur in NMS or orthostatic reactions, are recorded only by chance, if at all. Moreover, current ABPM technology, like long-term ECG monitoring, records only the momentary situation. Since syncopal episodes are so rare (even in "frequent" fainters), ABPM cannot then be counted on to document blood pressure during the syncope. Finally, current ABPM is too uncomfortable to use for many days in succession and usually too uncomfortable to be "transparent" to the autonomic nervous system.

Since the patient almost always remains asymptomatic during long-term blood pressure measurements, the record can in most cases only be scrutinized for surrogate end points, which might allow deductions about the cause of the syncope. This procedure has been accepted for long-term ECG, in spite of reasonable criticism. For example, a sudden asystole of >3 seconds is regarded (perhaps arguably) as adequate for the diagnosis of "arrythmogenic syncope" (if this is consistent with the medical history), indicating the necessity of pacemaker implantation (Figure 11.1). There are no corresponding parameters for long-term blood pressure measurements. So how large would blood pressure fluctuations within a 24-hour record have to be to allow the deduction of orthostatic dysregulation? As it has not been possible to define such parameters, long-term blood pressure measurements are used only sporadically in studies to clarify syncope and are not mentioned in the current guidelines. In a recently published trial, which investigated the current standard for management of syncope in 465 patients, ambulatory blood pressure management was performed in only a single patient [4].

Current ABPM is only clinically indicated for patients with postprandial hypotension (PPH) [5]. PPH is increasingly recognized as a common cause of syncope in elderly persons. ABPM has been used in research and clinical practice and has been proposed as the method of choice to evaluate fluctuations in blood pressure in patients with possible PPH [6]. Of course, the diagnosis of PPH is essentially made from the medical history. ABPM might nevertheless be helpful in documenting possible trigger mechanisms. However, there have not yet been any adequate studies on its possible role in monitoring therapeutic control.

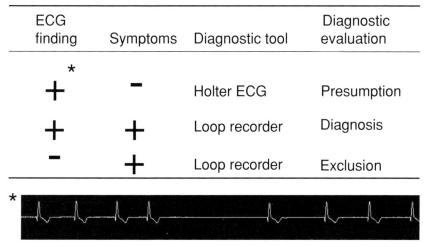

ECG finding	Symptoms	Diagnostic tool	Diagnostic evaluation
+*	−	Holter ECG	Presumption
+	+	Loop recorder	Diagnosis
−	+	Loop recorder	Exclusion

Figure 11.1 Correlation between ECG findings and symptoms during a spontaneous episode.

Future developments

The implantable loop recorder (ILR) is now essential for the diagnosis of unexplained syncope. It possesses the unrivaled advantage that an ECG is recorded at the time of syncope. It is then no longer necessary to argue on the basis of analogies, but a definitive diagnosis can be made (Figure 11.1).

On the other hand, the ILR measures only the ECG. For example, this is a disadvantage for patients thought to suffer from NMS, as it does not permit reliable conclusions about the actual relationships between cardioinhibitory and vasodepressive reactions. It would therefore be of great value if it were possible to perform long-term monitoring, with continuous recording of both the ECG and the blood pressure over several months. Systems of this sort are undergoing technological development. However, they cannot yet be used in the clinics and have not been scientifically validated.

Summary

Ambulatory blood pressure measurement is currently of secondary importance in syncope and TLOC, largely because of important technologic limitations. Consequently, as things stand, ABPM is dispensable for the diagnosis of orthostatic intolerance, as it only confirms what can be inferred from a carefully taken medical history. On the other hand, it could nevertheless become essential, especially in NMS, to the extent that it permits recognition of vasodepressor syncope and differentiation between the relative contribution of vasodepressor and cardioinhibitory mechanisms.

Clearly, it would be desirable to measure blood pressure during spontaneous syncope. Because of the rarity of syncopal events, ABPM, even over several days, is, like long-term ECG, of little use. An exception is PPH, which is predominantly observed in older people and which can be very reliably recorded by use of ABPM at specific times (i.e., meal times).

If it were possible to develop an ILR for the registration of not only the ECG but also the blood pressure, this would be a great step forward for the diagnosis of syncope. Because of the absence of important technical advances, we are a long way from the fulfillment of this dream.

References

1 Brignole M, Alboni P, Benditt DG, *et al*. Guidelines on management (diagnosis and treatment) of syncope—update 2004. Executive summary. *Eur Heart J* 2004;**25**:2054–72.

2 Moya A, Brignole M, Menozzi C, *et al*. Mechanism of syncope in patients with isolated syncope and in patients with tilt-positive syncope. *Circulation* 2001;**104**:1261–7.

3 O'Brien E, Coats A, Owens P, *et al*. Use and interpretation of ambulatory blood pressure monitoring: recommendations of the British Hypertension Society. *BMJ* 2000;**320**:1128–34.

4 Brignole M, Menozzi C, Bartoletti A, *et al*. A new management of syncope: prospective systematic guideline-based evaluation of patient referred urgently to general hospitals. *Eur Heart J* 2006;**27**:76–82.

5 Puisieux F, Bulckaen H, Fauchais AL, *et al*. Ambulatory blood pressure monitoring and postbrandial hypotension in elderly persons with falls or syncopes. *J Gerontol A Biol Sci Med Sci* 2000; **55**:M535–40.

6 Grodzicki T, Rajzer M, Fargard R; Systolic Hypertension in Europe (SYST-EUR) Trial Investigators. Ambulatory blood pressure monitoring and postbrandial hypotension in elderly patients with isolated systolic hypertension. *J Human Hypertens* 1998;**12**:161–5.

CHAPTER 12

Electrophysiologic testing: value and limitations in the transient loss of consciousness/syncope evaluation

Suneet Mittal

Introduction

Syncope is defined as the sudden loss of consciousness due to transient cerebral hypoperfusion (usually associated with the loss of postural tone) followed by a complete and rapid spontaneous recovery. It is a very common clinical problem. The overall incidence of a first report of syncope is 6.2/1000 person-years; the incidence rate increases with age, especially after the age of 70 [1]. The estimated 10-year cumulative incidence of syncope is 6%, and up to 22% of patient experience recurrent syncope [1].

The differential diagnosis of syncope is extensive. The evaluation of a patient presenting with syncope starts with the history and physical examination and almost always includes an electrocardiogram (ECG) and echocardiogram. An initial goal in the evaluation process is to distinguish cardiac from noncardiac causes of syncope.

Several historical features appear to be useful to identify a cardiac cause for syncope (also see Chapter 6). These include (1) syncope in the presence of severe structural heart disease, (2) syncope occurring while supine or during exertion, (3) syncope preceded by palpitations or accompanied by chest pain, and (4) syncope occurring in a patient with a family history of sudden death [2]. The aim of this chapter is to discuss the role and limitations of electrophysiologic (EP) testing in the evaluation of patients with suspected cardiac syncope due to an arrhythmia.

Bradyarrhythmias

Syncope due to a bradyarrhythmia can be related to sinus bradycardia resulting from sinus node dysfunction, or atrioventricular (AV) block resulting from AV node or His-Purkinje system dysfunction. Electrophysiological (EP) studies

Syncope and Transient Loss of Consciousness, 1st edition. Edited by David G Benditt *et al.*
© 2007 Blackwell Publishing, ISBN: 978-1-4051-7625-5.

are most useful when the patient's baseline ECG demonstrates sinus brady-cardia or conduction system disease. Specific high-risk abnormalities include asymptomatic sinus bradycardia (<50 bpm), sinoatrial block or sinus pause ≥3 seconds in the absence of negatively chronotropic medications, Mobitz I second-degree AV block, and bifascicular block (either left bundle branch block or right bundle branch block with left anterior or posterior fascicular block) [2]. In the setting of sinus bradycardia or evident AV conduction system disease, diagnostic findings at EP testing favoring a basis for syncope include (1) sinus bradycardia and a markedly prolonged corrected sinus node recovery time (CSRT ≫ 525 ms), or (2) bifascicular block and significant His-Purkinje system disease. The latter is reflected by a baseline His-ventricle (HV) interval of ≥100 milliseconds or the development of second- or third-degree His-Purkinje block during incremental atrial pacing or during infusion of ajmaline, pro-cainamide, or disopyramide (i.e., drugs used to further "stress" the conduction system) [2].

EP testing tends to have a high specificity but poor sensitivity for diagnosing patients at risk for symptomatic bradycardia. As a result, alternative diagnostic strategies are clearly needed. The most promising is the implantable loop recorder (ILR), a leadless "black box" (the current Reveal ILR from Medtronic Inc., Minneapolis, MN, is 61 × 19 × 8 mm, 8 cm^3, weight 17 g) with two self-contained electrodes that is implanted subcutaneously in a left parasternal location. The unit records a single-lead ECG continuously in 42-minute "loops" (either automatically or when activated by a patient) over its 14-month battery life (also see Chapter 10).

In a randomized study, a strategy of early loop recorder implantation was shown to be superior to a more conventional strategy of EP and tilt-table testing in making a definitive diagnosis (which was usually a form of bradycardia) in patients without structural heart disease presenting with syncope [3]. Furthermore, with the use of an implanted loop recorder, it has been possible to demonstrate that in a third of patients with bundle branch block (specifically, right bundle branch and fascicular block or left bundle branch block) recurrent syncope results from paroxysmal AV block, even though the EP study is "normal" [4].

Tachyarrhythmias

Ischemic cardiomyopathy

The yield of EP testing in patients with syncope is greatest in those with underlying structural heart disease, especially in those with an underlying ischemic cardiomyopathy. Sustained monomorphic ventricular tachycardia is inducible in 40% of these patients [5]. Inasmuch as these patients are at high risk for sudden cardiac death, an implantable cardioverter-defibrillator (ICD) is usually inserted, although syncope may not be prevented by this treatment alone. In contrast, induction of ventricular fibrillation, especially when achieved with triple ventricular extrastimuli, is not of prognostic significance [2, 6].

Within 15 months of ICD implantation, 40% of patients receive an appropriate therapy from the ICD for management of recurrent ventricular tachycardia or fibrillation [5]. The risk of recurrent events is greatest in patients with a prolonged QRS duration ($\geq$120 ms) [7]. Surprisingly, inducible patients, despite treatment with an ICD, have a higher overall mortality than noninducible patients [5]. Furthermore, studies using an implantable loop recorder have shown that syncope patients with underlying structural heart disease and a negative EP test have a more favorable outcome [8].

Despite the ability of EP testing to risk-stratify patients with an ischemic cardiomyopathy presenting with syncope, in the current era, EP testing is rarely performed in these patients. Since many of these patients have a significantly depressed left ventricular ejection fraction, they are candidates for ICD implantation based on the results of large-scale primary prevention ICD trials, such as Multicenter Automatic Defibrillator Implantation Trial II (MADIT-II) and Sudden Cardiac Death in Heart Failure Trial (SCD-HeFT). As a result, an investigation for the cause of syncope is often reserved for those who continue to experience syncope despite ICD implantation.

Nonischemic cardiomyopathy

An EP-guided approach is the most effective for patients with an ischemic cardiomyopathy. In patients with a nonischemic cardiomyopathy, the negative predictive value of EP testing is poor [9, 10]. Patients with a nonischemic cardiomyopathy whose left ventricular ejection fraction is less than 30% appear to have particularly high mortality risk [11]. Furthermore, patients treated with an ICD have a high likelihood of receiving appropriate therapies [12, 13]. Therefore, ICD implantation has been advocated in all of these patients who present with syncope, irrespective of the findings at EP testing. Interestingly, prospective data in this patient population are not available since ICD trials in patients with a nonischemic cardiomyopathy, such as Defibrillators in Nonischemic Cardiomyopathy Treatment Evaluation (DEFINITE) and Sudden Cardiac Death in Heart Failure Trial (SCD-HeFT), have specifically excluded patients with history of unexplained syncope.

Special populations

There are a number of genetic cardiovascular conditions that can be associated with syncope. These include conditions such as hypertrophic cardiomyopathy, arrhythmogenic right ventricular cardiomyopathy, Brugada syndrome, and congenital short or long QT-interval syndrome. There are no conclusive data to support the use of EP testing for risk stratification in patients with any of these conditions who present with syncope. As a result, ICD implantation is frequently performed in these patients. However, markers for better risk stratification are clearly needed; since these patients are generally young, the rate of appropriate ICD therapies over the short-term is relatively low, and the risk of system-related complications can often be unacceptably high.

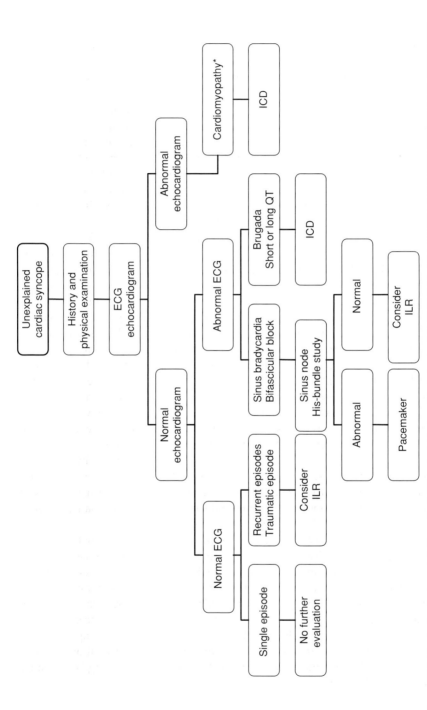

Figure 12.1 Generalized approach to the patient with unexplained cardiac syncope. ILR, implantable loop recorder; *, ischemic cardiomyopathy, nonischemic cardiomyopathy, hypertrophic cardiomyopathy, and arrhythmogenic right ventricular cardiomyopathy.

Conclusion

Syncope remains a common clinical problem. In most patients, a diagnosis can be readily made on the basis of the initial history and physical examination. When initial evaluation suggests cardiac syncope, the direction of further evaluation is driven by review of the patient's ECG and echocardiogram (Figure 12.1).

In patients with a normal ECG and no evidence of structural heart disease, syncope is usually the result of bradycardia. In younger patients, bradycardia is often secondary to a neurally-mediated phenomenon. In contrast, in older patients, it can be difficult to differentiate between a neurally-mediated event and an intrinsic sinus node dysfunction. Unfortunately, both EP and tilt-table testing have limited sensitivity in this patient population. As a result, implantation of an ILR is reasonable in some of these patients, especially in those in whom syncope is recurrent or associated with trauma.

In patients with an abnormal ECG (e.g., sinus bradycardia, first-degree or type I second-degree AV block, or fascicular block) but no structural heart disease, an EP study is reasonable to determine the need for pacing in the patient. The likelihood of ventricular tachyarrhythmias in this patient population is quite low. In the event in which EP testing is nondiagnostic, implantation of a loop recorder is also an appropriate step to take in this patient population. On the other hand, in patients with an ECG diagnostic for Brugada pattern or short or long QT-interval syndrome, ICD implantation is warranted.

In patients with structural heart disease, loosely defined as left ventricular dysfunction, ICD implantation is usually warranted on the basis of the underlying heart disease alone. It is important to recognize that EP testing, although rarely performed today in these patients, can effectively risk-stratify patients with an underlying ischemic cardiomyopathy. Patients with inducible monomorphic ventricular tachycardia remain at high risk despite ICD implantation. In contrast, in patients with a nonischemic cardiomyopathy or a high-risk genetic cardiovascular disorder (e.g., hypertrophic cardiomyopathy and arrhythmogenic right ventricular cardiomyopathy), EP testing has unproven diagnostic value. Although ICDs are usually implanted in these patients, better methods for risk stratification are clearly needed.

We have ushered in a new era in the evaluation of patients with syncope. Instead of asking, "Why did the patient faint?" we have been increasingly asking, "Does my patient merit treatment?" In that context, in patients with unexplained syncope and no structural heart disease, bradycardia is an important cause of syncope. When a pacemaker would be otherwise reasonable in these patients, a strategy of early loop recorder implantation should be considered. In contrast, in patients with unexplained syncope and underlying structural heart disease, ventricular tachycardia is an important consideration and ICD implantation is warranted. In either event, the role of EP testing is becoming increasingly limited.

References

1 Soteriades ES, Evans JC, Larson MG, *et al*. Incidence and prognosis of syncope. *N Engl J Med* 2002;**347**:878–85.

2 Brignole M, Alboni P, Benditt DG, *et al*.; Task Force on Syncope, European Society of Cardiology. Guidelines on management (diagnosis and treatment) of syncope—update 2004. Executive summary. *Eur Heart J* 2004;**25**:2054–72.

3 Krahn AD, Klein GJ, Yee R, Skanes AC. Randomized assessment of syncope trial: conventional diagnostic testing versus a prolonged monitoring strategy. *Circulation* 2001;**104**:46–51.

4 Brignole M, Menozzi C, Moya C, *et al*. Mechanism of syncope in patients with bundle branch block and negative electrophysiological tests. *Circulation* 2001;**104**:2045–50.

5 Mittal S, Iwai S, Stein KM, Markowitz SM, Slotwiner DJ, Lerman BB. Long-term outcome of patients with unexplained syncope treated with an electrophysiologic-guided approach in the implantable cardioverter-defibrillator era. *J Am Coll Cardiol* 1999;**34**:1082–9.

6 Mittal S, Hao SC, Iwai S, *et al*. Significance of inducible ventricular fibrillation in patients with coronary artery disease and unexplained syncope. *J Am Coll Cardiol* 2001;**38**:371–6.

7 Guttigoli AB, Wilner BF, Stein KM, *et al*. Usefulness of prolonged QRS duration to identify high-risk ischemic cardiomyopathy patients with syncope and inducible ventricular tachycardia. *Am J Cardiol* 2005;**95**:391–4.

8 Menozzi C, Brignole M, Garcia-Civera R, *et al*. Mechanism of syncope in patients with heart disease and negative electrophysiologic test. *Circulation* 2002;**105**:2741–5.

9 Brilakis ES, Shen WK, Hammill SC, *et al*. Role of programmed ventricular stimulation and implantable cardioverter defibrillators in patients with idiopathic dilated cardiomyopathy and syncope. *Pacing Clin Electrophysiol* 2001;**24**:1623–30.

10 Brilakis ES, Friedman PA, Maounis TN, *et al*. Programmed ventricular stimulation in patients with idiopathic dilated cardiomyopathy and syncope receiving implantable cardioverter-defibrillators: a case series and a systematic review of the literature. *Int J Cardiol* 2005;**98**:395–401.

11 Mittal S, Stephenson K, Stein KM, *et al*. Long-term outcome of patients with a non-ischemic cardiomyopathy and unexplained syncope [abstract]. *Pacing Clin Electrophysiol* 2000;**23**:560.

12 Knight BP, Goyal R, Pelosi F, *et al*. Outcome of patients with nonischemic dilated cardiomyopathy and unexplained syncope treated with an implantable cardioverter defibrillator. *J Am Coll Cardiol* 1999;**33**:1964–70.

13 Russo AM, Verdino R, Schorr C, *et al*. Occurrence of implantable defibrillator events in patients with syncope and nonischemic dilated cardiomyopathy. *Am J Cardiol* 201;**88**:1444–6.

CHAPTER 13

Intolerance to upright posture in autonomic failure and the postural tachycardia syndrome: assessment and treatment strategies

Christopher J Mathias

Introduction

Humans are bipeds and thus are exposed to gravitational (Newtonian) forces when upright. To overcome these effects, they have developed adaptive mechanisms—cardiovascular, hormonal, and neurogenic—to maintain blood pressure (BP) and heart rate (HR) so as to perfuse key organs adequately, especially while upright. Impairment of one or more of these factors can result in intolerance to the upright posture. This chapter will focus on orthostatic intolerance predominantly due to autonomic dysfunction in autonomic failure and the postural tachycardia syndrome (POTS).

Assessment

This is by a combination of clinical features and laboratory investigation.

Clinical features

There are many causes of autonomic failure [1]. Disease can affect the autonomic nervous system within the brain, spinal cord, periphery, or at multiple sites. There may be no specific cause, as in pure autonomic failure and multiple system atrophy. Common disorders include Parkinson's disease and diffuse Lewy body disease. Secondary causes include genetic disorders (familial dysautonomia), enzyme deficiencies (dopamine beta-hydroxylase deficiency), or complications of disease (diabetes mellitus and spinal cord injuries). A variety of drugs can impair autonomic function directly or by causing an autonomic neuropathy.

Syncope and Transient Loss of Consciousness, 1st edition. Edited by David G Benditt *et al.*
© 2007 Blackwell Publishing, ISBN: 978-1-4051-7625-5.

In autonomic failure, orthostatic (postural) hypotension is a cardinal feature. It can cause a variety of symptoms that mainly arise from underperfusion of organs: brain (dizziness, visual disturbances, transient cognitive deficits, and syncope [2, 3]), muscle (paracervical and suboccipital "coathanger" ache), and kidneys (oliguria). In some, nonspecific symptoms such as weakness, lethargy, and fatigue occur. In the elderly there may be falls of otherwise unknown etiology. Factors that worsen orthostatic hypotension in autonomic failure include nocturia (reducing intravascular fluid volume especially by the morning), prolonged recumbency, speed of positional change, cutaneous vasodilatation in hot weather and after a warm bath, ingestion of food and alcohol, physical exertion, and vasodilatatory drugs.

Autonomic failure affects all age groups and the prevalence rises with age. In autonomic failure there are often additional features involving other organs or systems affected by impaired autonomic control (bladder, gastrointestinal tract, genital in the male, sudomotor, or eye) or those resulting from associated disease (Parkinsonism or complications of diabetes mellitus).

In contrast, POTS is a disorder mainly affecting women between the ages of 20 and 50. Symptoms of orthostatic intolerance (light headedness and other manifestations of cerebral hypoperfusion) are often accompanied by palpitations. The symptoms disappear on sitting or lying down. There is a HR rise of over 30 bpm while upright, without a fall in BP. Palpitations are worse during exercise. Decompensation due to lack of physical activity may complicate the disorder. In some, hyperventilation and panic attacks may occur. Recent studies indicate that vasovagal syncope occurs in 25% of POTS [4]. This may be related to specific events, although it may occur without a recognized provoking cause; it is more likely to occur in the upright position. There are similarities with syndromes initially described by Da Costa and Lewis (soldier's heart or neurocirculatory asthenia), mitral valve prolapse, chronic fatigue syndrome, deconditioning following prolonged bed rest, and microgravity during spaceflight. Hypovolemia may contribute. It may follow a viral infection. There may be features of a partial autonomic neuropathy with lower limb denervation. Antibodies to autonomic ganglia have been related to the autonomic deficits. In a family with affected twins, a genetic basis has been proposed; there was mutation of the gene encoding the noradrenaline transporter system that may have accounted for the raised basal noradrenaline levels and hyperadrenergic state. There is an association with the joint hypermobility syndrome (Ehlers–Danlos III) [5].

Laboratory investigation

In orthostatic hypotension caused by autonomic failure, a multipronged investigation often is needed, ideally in an autonomic laboratory [6]. Initially, this would determine if autonomic function is normal or impaired. If latter, the degree of autonomic dysfunction and cause, along with the associated disorder, should be evaluated, as these aspects often determine the prognosis and aid anticipation of complications, thus modifying treatment strategies.

Autonomic function screening tests, in addition to head-up tilt testing to 60°, determine the site and extent of the cardiovascular autonomic abnormality. The responses to the Valsalva maneuver depend on the integrity of the entire baroreflex pathway. Stimuli that raise BP, such as isometric exercise, cold, and mental arithmetic, activate different afferent or central pathways, which then stimulate the sympathetic efferent outflow. The HR responses to postural change, deep breathing (sinus arrhythmia), and hyperventilation assess the function of cardiac parasympathetic efferent (vagus) pathways.

Ambulatory BP and HR recordings over a 24-hour period are of value, especially at home, in determining the effects of various stimuli in daily life and in monitoring the effects of therapy. Additional investigations may be needed to determine factors causing or contributing to orthostatic hypotension and syncope; these include the responses to food ingestion and exercise.

Similar assessments to those used in autonomic failure are of value in POTS.

Treatment strategies

Orthostatic intolerance in autonomic failure

Orthostatic hypotension may cause considerable disability, with the potential risk of serious injury. In neurogenic orthostatic hypotension, cure is less likely and long-term management needs to be considered. Management of associated nonneurogenic factors (such as resulting from fluid and blood loss) is essential, as they can exacerbate orthostatic hypotension. Nonpharmacologic measures are an essential component of management, even when drugs are used (Table 13.1a) [7]. No single drug can effectively mimic the actions of the sympathetic nervous system, and a multipronged drug approach often is needed (Table 13.1b) [8].

Orthostatic intolerance due to POTS

In POTS, similar nonpharmacologic measures should be introduced. Correcting hypovolemia by water drinking [9] and preventing contributory factors (such as hyperventilation) is important. A graded exercise program is helpful. The effects of associated disorders, such as the joint hypermobility syndrome that can result in substantial joint problems and pain, need to be addressed. When vasovagal syncope occurs, the treatment, especially when there is a low supine level of BP, should include dietary salt supplementation. In some with the cardioinhibitory form of vasovagal syncope, a cardiac demand pacemaker should be considered. Sympathetic activation techniques and antipooling measures that raise or prevent the fall in BP, especially in the presyncopal phase, often are of value.

The drug treatment of POTS differs from that of orthostatic hypotension. Fludrocortisone can help when the BP is low. Sympathomimetics that do not raise HR, such as midodrine, are of benefit. Cardioselective beta-adrenergic blockers may be helpful. Pyridostigmine has more recently been introduced as well [10].

Table 13.1 Some of the nondrug measures and drugs used in the management of orthostatic hypotension, especially in patients with autonomic failure syndromes (a); outline of the major actions by which a variety of drugs may reduce orthostatic hypotension (b).

(a)

Nonpharmacologic measures

To be avoided

Sudden head-up postural change (especially on waking)
Prolonged recumbency
Straining during micturition and defecation
High environmental temperature (including hot baths)
"Severe" exertion
Large meals (especially with refined carbohydrate)
Alcohol
Drugs with vasodepressor properties

To be introduced

Head-up tilt during sleep
Small frequent meals
High salt intake
Judicious exercise (including swimming)
Body positions and maneuvers

To be considered

Elastic stockings
Abdominal binders
Water ingestion

Pharmacologic measures

Starter drug—fludrocortisone
Sympathomimetics—ephedrine and midodrine
Specific targeting—octreotide, desmopressin, and erythropoietin

(b)

Reducing salt loss/plasma volume expansion

Mineralocorticoids (fludrocortisone)

Reducing nocturnal polyuria

V_2-receptor agonists (desmopressin)

Vasoconstriction

Sympathetic

On resistance vessels (ephedrine, midodrine, phenylephrine, noradrenaline, clonidine, tyramine with monoamine oxidase inhibitors, yohimbine, and L-dihydroxyphenylserine)
On capacitance vessels (dihydroergotamine)

Nonsympathomimetic

V_1-receptor agents (terlipressin)

Nicotinic acetylcholine receptor stimulation

anticholinesterase inhibitors (pyridostigmine)

Preventing vasodilatation

Prostaglandin synthetase inhibitors (indomethacin and flurbiprofen)
Dopamine receptor blockade (metoclopramide and domperidone)
β_2-adrenoceptor blockade (propranolol)

Preventing postprandial hypotension

Adrenosine receptor blockade (caffeine)
Peptide release inhibitors (somatostatin analog: octreotide)

Increasing cardiac output

Beta blockers with intrinsic sympathomimetic activity (pindolol and xamoterol)
Dopamine agonists (ibopamine)

Increasing red cell mass

Erythropoietin

Adapted from Mathias. Autonomic diseases: management. *J Neurol Neurosurg Psychiatry* 2003;**74**:iii42–7.

Conclusion

There is increasing recognition of autonomic disturbances as a cause of syncope and near syncope. The management includes careful assessment of factors aggravating the underlying disturbance (e.g., drugs). Treatment often necessitates a complex multipronged approach.

References

1 Mathias CJ. Orthostatic hypotension and orthostatic intolerance. In: DeGroot LJ, Jameson JL, de Kretser D, *et al.* (eds.), *Endocrinology*, 5th edn. Elsevier Saunders, Philadelphia PA, 2006: 2613–32.

2 Hunt K, Tachtsidis I, Bleasdale-Barr K, Elwell C, Mathias CJ, Smith M. Changes in cerebral oxygenation and haemodynamics during postural blood pressure changes in patients with autonomic failure. *Physiol Meas* 2006;**27**:777–85.

3 Mathias CJ, Mallipeddi R, Bleasdale-Barr K. Symptoms associated with orthostatic hypotension in pure autonomic failure and multiple system atrophy. *J Neurol* 1999;**246**: 893–8.

4 Hajdinjak M, Harris S, Corridan M, *et al.* Diagnosing postural tachycardia syndrome— head up tilt or standing? *Clin Auton Res* 2006;**16**:156–7.

5 Gazit Y, Nahir AM, Grahame R, Jacob G. Dysautonomia in the joint hypermobility syndrome. *Am J Med* 2003;**115**:33–40.

6 Mathias CJ. Role of autonomic evaluation in the diagnosis and management of syncope. *Clin Auton Res* 2004;**14**:S1, 45–54.

7 Mathias CJ. Autonomic diseases management. *J Neurol Neurosurg Psychiatry* 2003;**74**:iii42– 7.

8 Schroeder C, Vernino S, Birkenfeld A, *et al.* Plasma exchange for primary autoimmune autonomic failure. *N Engl J Med* 2005;**353**:1585–90.

9 Mathias CJ, Young TM. Water drinking in the management of orthostatic intolerance due to orthostatic hypotension, vasovagal syncope and the postural tachycardia syndrome. *Eur J Neurol* 2004;**11**:613–19.

10 Gales BJ, Gales MA. Pyridostigmine in the treatment of orthostatic intolerance. *Ann Pharmacother* 2007;**41**:314–18.

CHAPTER 14

Improving tolerance to upright posture: current status of tilt-training and other physical maneuvers

Hugo Ector, Tony Reybrouck

Neurally-mediated syncope is the result of a sudden imbalance between orthostatic tolerance and gravitational stress. It occurs with or without prodromal symptoms. In the case of an acute episode with premonitory symptoms, physical maneuvers initiated by the affected individual may prevent frank syncope. However, the ultimate goal of treatment is freedom from syncope. In this respect, tilt-training has been introduced as a means of improving orthostatic tolerance for motivated patients with recurrent neurally-mediated vasovagal syncope.

Physical maneuvers

In a remarkable case report, Wieling, van Lieshout, and Leeuwen [1] described a series of maneuvers that help to reduce the symptoms of severe orthostatic hypotension: squatting, standing with the head bent and with contracted abdominal muscles, leg crossing, putting a foot on a chair, bending over as if to tie one's shoes, sitting in the knee–chest position, and abdominal compression.

In terms of the mechanism of potential benefits offered by the physical countermaneuver techniques, a number of issues are pertinent. For example, bending forward shortens the hydrostatic height difference between the heart and the brain. Leg crossing and abdominal compression enhance venous return from the lower part of the body.

van Dijk *et al.* [2] reported the hemodynamic effects of leg crossing and skeletal muscle tensing during free standing in patients with vasovagal syncope. Eighty-eight patients diagnosed with vasovagal syncope applied leg crossing after a 5-minute free-standing period. Fifty-four of these patients also applied tensing of leg and abdominal muscles. Leg crossing produced a significant rise in cardiac output, thereby increasing mean arterial pressure. Muscle tensing created an additional increase in cardiac output and mean

Syncope and Transient Loss of Consciousness, 1st edition. Edited by David G Benditt *et al.*
© 2007 Blackwell Publishing, ISBN: 978-1-4051-7625-5.

arterial pressure. The rise in blood pressure during leg crossing was larger in the elderly.

In another study, Brignole *et al.* [3] proposed arm counterpressure maneuvers to abort impending vasovagal syncope: isometric handgrip and isometric arm contraction. In an acute tilt-table study, handgrip was administered for 2 minutes, starting at the time of onset of symptoms of impending syncope. The patients were trained to self-administer arm-tensing treatment as soon as symptoms of impending syncope occurred. The treatment was performed in 95 of 97 episodes of impending syncope and was successful in 94 out of 95. In the active arm, 63% of patients became asymptomatic versus 11% in the control arm; conversely, only 5% of patients developed syncope versus 47% in the control arm.

In one report [4], the techniques of "squatting" or "leg crossing with muscle tensing" were more effective than handgrip as acute physical countermaneuvers.

Tilt-training

Tilt-training is a technique that has been devised with the goal of reducing orthostatic intolerance, thereby diminishing susceptibility to neurally-mediated and orthostatic faints. Conceptually, over time, tilt-training forces the autonomic nervous system to more effectively and appropriately control vascular tone; this is accomplished by exposing the patient to prolonged periods of quiet upright posture. In a recent study, Gajek *et al.* have analyzed the complex influence of tilt-training on the activation of the autonomic nervous system [5].

In Leuven, for patients with recurrent neurally-mediated syncope, we organize a daily in-hospital tilt-table test (60° inclination). Every test is continued until syncope, symptoms of orthostatic intolerance, or until completion of a maximum duration of 45 minutes. We do not use pharmacologic provocation. The patient is discharged from the hospital after two consecutive negative tests. The therapeutic impact of repeated tilt-table testing is maintained by continued standing training at home. We advise standing and leaning with the upper back against a wall and the feet 15 cm away from the wall. The patients are instructed not to move their feet and to maintain a static position. Reading a newspaper, radio listening, and watching TV are allowed. Supervision by a family member is recommended, certainly for the first home sessions. The standing session requires a safe place without risk of injury. It has to be terminated at the occurrence of the first symptom. After discharge from the hospital, we recommend two standing sessions per day of 30 minutes each.

Six weeks later, a new tilt-table test is performed during an outpatient visit. If this test is negative (normal duration of 45 min), the patient is advised to continue home therapy, but the frequency of standing sessions is reduced to one per day. Other outpatient clinic visits with control tilt-table tests are planned after 3 months, 6 months, and 1 year. After 1 year of standing train-ing, for asymptomatic patients, the frequency of tilt-training sessions can be reduced.

We have reported on repeated tilt-table testing in 222 patients with recurrent neurally-mediated syncope [6]. In 54% of the patients, the second consecutive tilt-table test was already negative. For an additional 21%, the third session was the first negative test. Only 25% of our patients remained symptomatic for three or more sessions. Finally, a negative tilt-table test could be obtained for every patient. For highly symptomatic patients, adhering to our treatment protocol, we have obtained excellent long-term results [7, 8].

In an interesting report, standing training was considered not to be effective in reducing tilt-table testing positivity [9]. In this study, only a minority of the patients performed all the programmed sessions. Patients were instructed to start standing training at home. There was no initial repeated tilt-table testing. The rationale for our initial in-hospital tilt-table testing is that for very symp-tomatic patients, it restores orthostatic tolerance in a few days. It adds to the motivation to continue standing training at home. Nowadays, in some cases, we also prescribe immediate out-of-hospital standing training, provided that adequate supervision by a well-informed family member is available.

We concur with our colleagues [9] that tilt-training appears to be a feasible treatment only for highly motivated patients. In our long-term follow-up [8], the experience is that patients adapt the standing training schedule to their own needs. Some intensify standing training by increasing the number of sessions or by increasing the duration of sessions. Others reduce the standing training program and resume it when symptoms recur.

Other authors [10] suggest that successful results can also be obtained with a transient tilt-training program. The easier performance and high effectiveness rate would most likely result in a more frequent utilization of tilt-training. Their patients followed a tilt-training program with two phases: in-hospital tilt-training until three consecutive negative tests and home exercises with standing against a wall. The home exercises were continued for a maximum of 2 months. After this training program, the patients did not receive any treatment. At the end of the follow-up period, 81% of the patients were free from recurrent syncope. The easier training program favored the acceptance rate of the training program.

Conclusion

Recent experience suggests that physical countermaneuvers have an important role to play in the long-term treatment of neurally-mediated vasovagal syn-cope. Certain maneuvers such as leg crossing and muscle tensing are appropri-ate for ameliorating acute episodes. In the longer term, however, tilt-training may be effective for reducing susceptibility to recurrent neurally-mediated faints.

References

1 Wieling W, van Lieshout JJ, van Leeuwen AM. Physical maneuvers that reduce postural hypotension in autonomic failure. *Clin Auton Res* 1993;**3**:57–65.

2 van Dijk N, de Bruin IGJ, Gisolf J, *et al*. Hemodynamic effects of leg crossing and skeletal muscle tensing during free standing in patients with vasovagal syncope. *J Appl Physiol* 1998;**98**:584–90.

3 Brignole M, Croci F, Menozzi C, *et al*. Isometric arm counter-pressure maneuvers to abort impending vasovagal syncope. *J Am Coll Cardiol* 2002;**40**:2053–9.

4 Kim KH, Cho JG, Lee KO, *et al* Usefulness of physical maneuvers for prevention of vasovagal syncope. *Circ J* 2005;**69**:1084–8.

5 Gajek J, Zysko D, Halawa B, Mazurek W. Influence of tilt training on activation of the autonomic nervous system in patients with vasovagal syncope. *Acta Cardiol* 2006;**61**:123–8.

6 Ector H, Willems R, Heidbüchel H, Reybrouck T. Repeated tilt testing in patients with tilt-positive neurally mediated syncope. *Europace* 2005;**7**:628–33.

7 Reybrouck T, Heidbüchel H, Van De Werf F, Ector H. Tilt training: a treatment for malignant and recurrent neurocardiogenic syncope. *Pacing Clin Electrophysiol* 2000;**23**:493–8.

8 Reybrouck T, Heidbüchel H, Van De Werf F, Ector H. Long-term follow-up results of tilt training therapy in patients with recurrent neurocardiogenic syncope. *Pacing Clin Electrophysiol* 2002;**25**:144–6.

9 Foglia-Manzillo G, Giada F, Gaggioli G, *et al*. Efficacy of tilt training in the treatment of neurally mediated syncope. *Europace* 2004;**6**:199–204.

10 Kinay O, Yazici M, Nazli C, *et al*. Tilt training for recurrent neurocardiogenic syncope: effectiveness, patient compliance, and scheduling the frequency of training sessions. *Jpn Heart J* 2004;**45**:833–43.

CHAPTER 15

Syncope in patients with bundle-branch block and other conduction system abnormalities

Angel Moya

In the patient being evaluated for syncope, the presence of intraventricular conduction abnormalities on baseline electrocardiogram is a strong marker of an arrhythmic origin of the faints.

In the case of alternating right and left bundle-branch block or right bundle branch block with alternating left anterior and left posterior fascicular block, the findings must be considered "diagnostic" of the cause of syncope (i.e., paroxysmal atrioventricular (AV) block) and no further tests need be performed. These patients should be treated with a pacemaker. In most cases, however, the mere presence of an abnormality is not sufficient to confidently establish a diagnosis. A carefully directed further evaluation is needed.

Bifascicular bundle-branch block

Several authors have shown that between 32% and 71% of patients with syncope and bifascicular bundle-branch block (BBBB) have structural heart diseases [1, 2]. For this reason, in these patients, a full cardiac evaluation, usually including an echocardiogram, should be performed in order to assess the presence and severity of structural heart disease.

The most frequent etiology of syncope in patients with syncope and BBBB is paroxysmal AV block. However, AV block is not the only potential cause of syncope in these individuals. Ventricular tachyarrhythmias are also a consideration and, at one point in time, were thought to be the more important cause. In addition, these patients can also develop, as in the general population, neurally-mediated reflex syncope (i.e., vasovagal syncope, carotid sinus syndrome, etc.).

In 1982, McAnulty et al. showed that up to 17% of patients with syncope and BBBB developed AV block at follow-up [3]. In 1983, Scheinman et al. studied 401 patients with syncope and BBBB, in whom an intracavitary

Syncope and Transient Loss of Consciousness, 1st edition. Edited by David G Benditt *et al.*
© 2007 Blackwell Publishing, ISBN: 978-1-4051-7625-5.

electrophysiologic study (EPS) was performed. During a follow-up of 30 months, AV block appeared in 3.5% of those patients who had a baseline His-ventricle (HV) interval <70 ms, 12% of those who had an HV interval between 70 and 100 ms, and 25% of those with HV interval longer than 100 ms [4], suggesting that the longer the HV interval, the greater the risk of developing AV block. Other authors have shown that in those patients with normal baseline HV interval, the presence of an infra-His block during incremental atrial pacing [5], or an abnormal lengthening of HV interval after intravenous administration of class IC antiarrhythmic drugs (or class IA where parenteral IC drugs are not available) [6], identified a subgroup of patients at higher risk of developing AV block subsequently.

Electrophysiologic testing

The data cited above suggest that in patients with BBBB and syncope of unknown origin, an EPS is indicated for further evaluation [7]. The study protocol of EPS in these patients must include evaluation of sinus node function, measurement of intracavitary AV conduction intervals, and if they are normal, progressive atrial pacing and intravenous administration of class IC or IA antiarrhythmic drugs. In addition, programmed supraventricular and ventricular stimulation should be performed in order to test for susceptibility for supraventricular or ventricular arrhythmias.

Unfortunately, while EPS may be helpful, it is not without limitations. The absence of an abnormal finding at EPS does not exclude an arrhythmic etiology of syncope as evidenced by the International Study on Syncope of Uncertain Etiology (ISSUE) findings [8]. In one component of the multicenter, multi-faceted ISSUE study, an implantable loop recorder (ILR) was implanted in syncope patients with BBBB and both a normal EPS and a preserved left ventricular ejection fraction. Paroxysmal AV block was documented in up to 50% of those who had recurrent syncope. In addition, 25% of the patients showed an asystolic pause preceded by progressive sinus bradycardia, strongly suggestive of a neurally-mediated reflex origin to the bradyarrhythmia and syncope. These data confirm that a negative EPS does not exclude an arrhythmia as a cause of syncope and that a neurally-mediated reflex syncope can also be present in patients with BBBB.

In brief, and consistent with the current European Society of Cardiology Syncope Guidelines, in all syncope patients with BBBB and in whom the etiology of syncope has not been established during initial evaluation, a complete cardiac evaluation designed to evaluate the presence of structural heart disease is recommended. Those in whom structural heart disease can be considered related to the etiology of syncope must be treated appropriately for the findings. However, despite the identification of underlying structural disease, the findings may not fully account for the syncope symptoms, and additional testing may be essential. EPS may be needed to assess for sinus node function (i.e., susceptibility to sinus pauses or arrest or bradycardia-tachycardia syndrome), AV conduction disease, and inducibility of supraventricular or ventricular arrhythmias. However, EPS findings must be carefully considered to make sure that they are consistent with the clinical circumstances. For example, in one study [9], in which bradyarrhythmias were known to be the cause of syncope (21 syncopal patients with known symptomatic AV block or sinus pauses), electrophysiologic testing correctly identified only 3 of 8 patients with documented sinus pauses (sensitivity 37.5%) and 2 of 13 patients with documented AV block (sensitivity 15.4%). On the other hand, other abnormalities, not known to have occurred spontaneously in these individuals, were often induced during EPS.

Treatment

For patients with data suggestive of bradyarrhythmia, either sinus node dysfunction or AV abnormal His-Purkinje system, pacemaker therapy is most likely indicated. In those with inducible supraventricular or ventricular tachycardia, treatment must focus on arrhythmia suppression. Ideally, radiofrequency catheter ablation should be undertaken if the rhythm can be targeted by that modality. However, drugs may be necessary in many cases. In patients with depressed left ventricular function, an implantable cardioverter-defibrillator (ICD) must be considered mainly due to the increased risk of sudden death. However, ICDs may not prevent syncope in these individuals; concomitant drug or ablation strategies are often needed.

In patients with preserved left ventricular function and in whom EPS has been negative or inconclusive, an ILR can be implanted and followed until first syncopal recurrence. Some investigators are beginning to use ILRs even earlier in the syncope assessment strategy; they argue that despite higher initial cost (due to the cost of both device and the implantation), the ultimate cost per diagnosis is in fact less than that with the conventional investigation approach.

Conclusion

The European Society of Cardiology Syncope Guidelines [10] serve as a detailed resource for identifying the most effective strategy for evaluation of syncope patients with overt or suspected conduction system disease. In this chapter we have emphasized current concepts, in particular the need to fully assess the status of underlying heart disease in syncope patients and the value of implantable monitors as an important tool to establish with certainty causal diagnoses.

References

1 Click R, Gersh B, Sugrue D, *et al*. Role of invasive electrophysiologic testing in patients with symptomatic bundle branch block. *Am J Cardiol* 1987;**59**:817–23.

2 Twidale N, Tonkin AM. Clinical electrophysiology study in patients with syncope of undetermined etiology. *Aust N Z J Med* 1987;**17**:512–17.

3 McAnulty JH, Rahimtoola SH, Murphy E, *et al*. Natural history of "high risk" bundle branch block: final report of a prospective study. *N Engl J Med* 1982;**307**:137–43.

4 Scheinman MM, Peters RW, Sauvé MJ, *et al*. Value of the H-Q interval in patients with bundle branch block and the role of prophylactic permanent pacing. *Am J Cardiol* 1982;**50**:1316–22.

5 Petrac D, Radic B, Birtic K, *et al*. Prospective evaluation of infrahisian second-degree AV block induced by atrial pacing in the presence of chronic bundle branch block and syncope. *Pacing Clin Electrophysiol* 1996;**19**:679–87.

6 Englund A, Bergfeldt L, Rosenqvist M. Pharmacological stress testing of the His-Purkinje system in patients with bifascicular block. *Pacing Clin Electrophysiol* 1998;**21**:1979–87.

7 Brignole M, Alboni P, Benditt DG, *et al*.; Task Force on Syncope, European Society of Cardiology. Guidelines on management (diagnosis and treatment) of syncope—update 2004. Executive summary. *Eur Heart J* 2004;**25**(22):2054–72.

8 Menozzi C, Brignole M, Garcia-Civera R, *et al*.; International Study on Syncope of Uncertain Etiology (ISSUE) Investigators. Mechanism of syncope in patients with heart disease and negative electrophysiologic test. *Circulation* 2002;**105**(23):2741–5.

9 Fujimura O, Yee R, Klein GJ, *et al*. The diagnostic sensitivity of electrophysiologic testing in patients with syncope caused by bradycardia. *N Engl J Med* 1989;**321**:1703–7.

10 Brignole M, Alboni P, Benditt DG, *et al*. Task force on syncope, European Society of Cardiology. Guidelines on Management (diagnosis and treatment) of syncope—update 2004. Executive summary. *Europace* 2004;**6**:467–537.

PART 3

Specific conditions

Treatment strategies in neurally-mediated reflex syncope: effectiveness of drugs, pacing, and physical maneuvers

Richard Sutton

Treatment of neurally-mediated reflex syncope begins with reassurance of the patient combined with explanation of the trigger mechanisms and its benign nature. The patient, however, should be warned about the potential for physical injury and how best it can be avoided. Secondly, the patient must be encouraged to consume large quantities of fluid and minimize caffeine, and those who are hypotensive (or at least not hypertensive) should take an increased quantity of salt.

Physical maneuvers

Paying attention to the situations in which syncope is likely to occur and to physical warnings from the body, such as nausea, sweating, air hunger, and dizziness, can allow the patient to take protective action, such as certain physical countermaneuvers, which may avert syncope. Application of physical maneuvers at this stage [1, 2] can make an important contribution to the prevention of syncope. These are practical measures that can be performed by a large majority of those experiencing neurally-mediated syncope; some of these are unproven by clinical trial but none represents a great imposition on, or danger to, the patient. The recently published multicenter Physical Counterpressure Maneuvers Trial (PC Trial) [3] compared the impact of usual therapy plus physical maneuvers ($n = 106$) with usual therapy alone ($n = 117$) in patients (38 ± 15 yr of age) who had recurrent vasovagal syncope and recognizable warning symptoms (see also Chapter 27). Actuarial recurrence-free survival was better in the treatment group (log-rank $p < 0.018$), resulting in a relative risk reduction of 39% (95% CI 11–53).

Syncope and Transient Loss of Consciousness, 1st edition. Edited by David G Benditt *et al.*
© 2007 Blackwell Publishing, ISBN: 978-1-4051-7625-5.

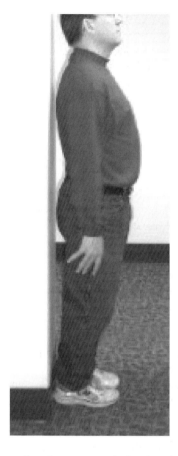

Figure 16.1 Tilt-training technique for home application is depicted. Patient stands without leg movement for prescribed periods of time. The duration of "stand time" is slowly increased over many weeks in an attempt to improve upright postural tolerance. Note that the floor is carpeted, there are no sharp objects nearby, and the wall behind the patient is used to diminish the risk of falling backward (not for physical support). (Courtesy, Cardiac Arrhythmia Center, University of Minnesota, Minneapolis, MN.)

Another approach that has been well studied [4, 5] is that of tilt or standing training. Patients may begin by being tilted on consecutive days until syncope does not occur: they then have to stand at home for 30 minutes, once or twice per day. Often in clinical practice the formal tilt portion as described by Reybrouck *et al.* [4] is omitted. Patients are taught to initiate standing training at home (Figure 16.1). Usually this is done with the individual standing with his or her back near a wall to prevent falling backward. The duration of standing is progressively but slowly increased over several weeks.

Reybrouck *et al.* [4] have had considerable success preventing vasovagal syncope recurrences with the tilt-training technique (see also Chapter 14 in this book). The benefits have also been reproduced by at least one other group in Japan [5]. However, a report from Italy was less favorable [6].

Drug therapy

Drugs have received much attention in the literature for treatment of neurally-mediated syncope over many years, but with the advent of clinical trials only one has survived this level of scrutiny. Beta blockers were once popular perhaps based on the finding of increased epinephrine prior to tilt-induced syncope [7]. Multiple trials of beta blockers have all been negative (see Sheldon *et al.* [8]), with one exception [9] where follow-up was short and success was determined by response to repeat tilt-table testing—a now discredited means of assessment because of the lack of reproducibility of the test. The most important beta-blocker trial in recent years is the Prevention of Syncope Trial (POST) [8] that failed to show benefit in terms of prevention of recurrence of syncope.

Etilefrine [10], a modest alpha and beta agonist, was evaluated in the Vasovagal Syncope International Study (VASIS) and did not prove effective. Similarly, the widely used mineralocorticoid fludrocortisone has not shown favorably under the rigor of a clinical trial [11]. However, clinical experience still favors fludrocortisone, suggesting that additional evaluation of this approach remains warranted (the POST 2 Trial is currently ongoing to test fludrocortisone in a double-blind randomized controlled manner). One other drug, midodrine, an alpha agonist that may have particular constrictive properties on the splanchnic venous bed, has evidence supporting its usefulness in more than one trial [12–14]. This drug, however, may precipitate urinary retention in older males because of its alpha-agonistic effect on urinary outflow. Additionally, as with any vasoconstrictor, it has the potential of aggravating hypertension. Thus, while helpful, it must be used with caution. A selective serotonin reuptake inhibitor has been found helpful in only one trial [15] that showed reduced recurrence of syncope in a group of 30 patients on active medication compared with a similar number on placebo: reproduction of these results is awaited. In summary, drugs have a limited role in the management of this condition and must be combined with physical maneuvers, fluid and salt increase, and education. This combined approach is not perfect, and in particular the long-term management by these agents is complicated in a variety of settings, including older men, hypertensive patients, and women who may be considering to become pregnant.

Pacemakers

Vasovagal syncope

Pacing has been thought valuable in the treatment of neurally-mediated syncope, especially in those who experience cardioinhibition (i.e., asystole or marked bradycardia) at the time. Initial trials [16–18] compared pacing with either continuation of existing medical treatment, no treatment, or, in one study, with atenolol [18] in which pacing looked favorable in each case. However, later studies of patients, all of whom had pacemaker implants but in whom pacing was "inactive" in a portion [19, 20], were not convincing of any benefit. Patient selection for these trials was loosely based on tilt-induced cardioinhibition, but recent work has shown that collapse patterns on tilt-table testing may not be the same as those during spontaneous attacks [21].

The International Study on Syncope of Uncertain Etiology 2 (ISSUE-2) [22] attempted to clarify the potential for better selection of patients who might benefit from pacing therapy. This study selected patients (over the age of 40) on the basis of spontaneously occurring asystole during neurally-mediated syncope. ISSUE-2 was only a registry (i.e., not a randomized trial) but in follow-up for 1 year in two groups (paced and unpaced), pacing appeared to have convincing benefits. The ISSUE-3 [23] trial is currently in progress, and it has the goal of more definitively determining whether pacing has merit in some patients. ISSUE-3 has the same selection criteria as ISSUE-2 but all patients who show asystole during a spontaneous attack recorded by an implanted loop recorder (ILR) will receive dual-chamber pacemakers; half will be randomized to ODO mode (in essence the pacemaker is turned "OFF") and the other half to active pacing. The trial results are expected in 2009.

In conclusion, pacing is as yet an unproven treatment in neurally-mediated reflex vasovagal syncope but consideration can be given today to the older patient with neurally-mediated syncope whose attacks are severe, with little or no warning, and in whom asystole has been documented during an attack.

Carotid sinus syndrome

The role of pacing in carotid sinus syndrome (CSS) is considered established, although most reports of its efficacy are anecdotal [24, 25] and only one small trial has been performed [26]. Likewise the role of drugs in CSS has been shown only to be effective as support for pacing with no drug alone having benefit in the cardioinhibitory type. In contrast, the vasodepressor form may benefit from midodrine [12].

Impact on future treatment guidelines

The possible influence of most recent work on future practice guidelines for management of neurally-mediated syncope may impact the levels of approach to management, as seen in Table 16.1. Secondly, recent studies strongly support an increased emphasis on the value of physical countermeasures [1, 2], a concept that has not previously been a focus of treatment recommendations. Thirdly, conventional thinking related to use of drug therapy in vasovagal syncope needs reappraisal. Recent studies regarding pharmacologic treatment for control of neurally-mediated syncope have been largely negative. Lastly, a new

Table 16.1 Treatment strategy for neurally-mediated syncope.

Level	Treatment	Patients
1		All
a	Explanation and reassurance	
b	Fluid and salt increase, and caffeine decrease	
c	Attention to warnings	
d	Physical countermeasures	
2	Standing (tilt) training	Any
3	Drugs—midodrine	Severely affected females
4	Pacing	Severely affected older patients

approach to the selection of patients for pacing may validate an effective role for this treatment in older, severely affected sufferers from neurally-mediated syncope who exhibit asystole or marked bradycardia during spontaneous attacks, as documented on ECG recordings from an ILR or other ambulatory ECG system.

Conclusion

Apart from CSS in which cardiac pacing remains the key treatment strategy, recent trends (based on a growing number of studies as well as clinical experience) for treatment of neurally-mediated vasovagal syncope tend to favor renewed emphasis on education, explanation, and reassurance backed by physical measures (i.e., leg crossing and tilt training). Resort to drug therapy or pacing is only to be considered in severely affected patients.

References

1 Krediet P, van Dijk N, Linzer M, *et al*. Management of vasovagal syncope controlling or aborting faints by leg crossing and muscle tensing. *Circulation* 2002;**106**:1684–9.

2 Podoleanu C, Maggi R, Brignole M, *et al*. Lower limb and abdominal compression bandages prevent progressive orthostatic hypotension in the elderly: a randomized placebo-controlled study. *J Am Coll Cardiol* 2006;**48**:1425–32.

3 van Dijk N, Quartieri F, Blanc JJ, *et al*. Effectiveness of physical counterpressure maneuvers in preventing vasovagal syncope: the Physical Counterpressure Manoeuvres Trial (PC-Trial). *J Am Coll Cardiol* 2006;**48**:1652–78.

4 Reybrouck T, Heidbuchel H, Van Der Werf F, *et al*. Long-term follow-up results of tilt training therapy in patients with recurrent neurocardiogenic syncope. *Pacing Clin Electrophysiol* 2002;**25**:1441–6.

5 Abe H, Kondo S, Kohshi K, *et al*. Usefulness of orthostatic self-training for the prevention of neurocardiogenic syncope. *Pacing Clin Electrophysiol* 2002;**25**:1454.

6 Foglia-Manzillo G, Giada F, Gaggioli G, *et al*. Efficacy of tilt training in the treatment of neurally mediated syncope: a randomized study. *Europace* 2004;**6**:199–204.

7 Fitzpatrick A, Williams T, Ahmed R, Lightman S, Bloom SR, Sutton R. Echocardiographic and endocrine changes during vasovagal syncope induced by prolonged head-up tilt. *Eur J Cardiac Pacing Electrophysiol* 1992;**2**:121–8.

8 Sheldon R, Connolly S, Rose S, *et al.*; POST Investigators. Prevention of Syncope Trial (POST): a randomized, placebo-controlled study of metoprolol in the prevention of vasovagal syncope. *Circulation* 2006;**113**:1164–70.

9 Mahananda N, Bhuripanyo K, Kangkagate C, *et al*. Randomized double-blind placebo-controlled trial oral atenolol in patients with unexplained syncope and positive upright tilt table results. *Am Heart J* 1995;**130**:1250–3.

10 Raviele A, Brignole M, Sutton R, *et al*. Effect of etilefrine in preventing syncopal recurrence in patients with vasovagal syncope: a double-blind, randomized, placebo-controlled trial. The Vasovagal Syncope International Study. *Circulation* 1999;**99**:1452–7.

11 Salim MA, Di Sessa TG. Effectiveness of fludrocortisone and salt in preventing syncope recurrence in children: a double-blind, placebo-controlled, randomized trial. *J Am Coll Cardiol* 2005;**45**:484–8.

12 Ward CR, Gray JC, Gilroy JJ, *et al.* Midodrine: a role in the management of neurocardiogenic syncope. *Heart* 1998;**79**:45–9.

13 Perez-Lugones A, Schwelkert R, Pavia S, *et al.* Usefulness of midodrine in patients with severely symptomatic neurocardiogenic syncope: a randomised controlled study. *J Cardiovasc Electrophysiol* 2001;**12**:935–8.

14 Moore A, Watts M, Sheehy T, Hartnett A, Clinch D, Lyons D. Treatment of vasodepressor carotid sinus syndrome with midodrine: a randomized, controlled pilot study. *J Am Geriatr Soc* 2005;**53**:114–18.

15 Di Girolamo E, Di Iorio C, Sabatini G, *et al.* Effects of paroxetine hydrochloride, a selective serotonin reuptake inhibitor, on refractory vasovagal syncope: a randomised, double blind placebo-controlled study. *J Am Coll Cardiol* 1999;**33**:1227–30.

16 Connolly SJ, Sheldon R, Roberts RS, *et al.*; Vasovagal Pacemaker Study Investigators. The North American vasovagal pacemaker study [VPS]: a randomised trial of permanent cardiac pacing for the prevention of vasovagal syncope. *J Am Coll Cardiol* 1999;**33**:16–20.

17 Sutton R, Brignole M, Menozzi C, *et al.*; The Vasovagal Syncope International Study [VASIS] Investigators. Dual-chamber pacing in the treatment of neurally mediated tilt-positive cardioinhibitory syncope: pacemaker vs no therapy. A multi-center randomized study. *Circulation* 2000;**102**:294–9.

18 Ammirati F, Colivicchi F, Santini M, *et al.* Permanent cardiac pacing versus medical treatment for the prevention of recurrent vasovagal syncope: a multicenter, randomised, controlled trial. *Circulation* 2001;**104**:52–7.

19 Connolly SJ, Sheldon R, Thorpe KE, *et al.*, for the VPS II Investigators. Pacemaker therapy for prevention of syncope in patients with recurrent severe vasovagal syncope: second Vasovagal Pacemaker Study [VPS II]. *JAMA* 2003;**289**:2224–9.

20 Raviele A, Giada F, Menozzi C, *et al.* The vasovagal syncope and pacing trial [SYNPACE]: a randomised, double-blind, placebo-controlled study of permanent pacing for treatment of recurrent tilt-induced vasovagal syncope. *Eur Heart J* 2004;**25**:1741–8.

21 Moya A, Brignole M, Menozzi C, *et al.* Mechanism of syncope in patients with isolated syncope and in patients with tilt positive syncope. *Circulation* 2001;**104**:1261–7.

22 Brignole M, Sutton R, Menozzi C, *et al.* Early application of an implantable loop recorder allows a mechanism-based effective therapy in patients with recurrent suspected neurally-mediated syncope. *Eur Heart J* 2006;**27**:1085–92.

23 The Steering Committee of the ISSUE 3 Study. International Study on Syncope of Uncertain Aetiology 3 [ISSUE 3]: pacemaker therapy for patients with asystolic neurally-mediated syncope. Rationale and study design. *Europace* 2007;**9**:25–30.

24 Morley CA, Perrins EJ, Grant PL, *et al.* Carotid sinus syncope treated by pacing: analysis of persistent symptoms and role of atrio-ventricular sequential pacing. *Br Heart J* 1982;**47**:411–18.

25 Madigan NP, Flaker GC, Curtis JJ, *et al.* Carotid sinus hypersensitivity: beneficial effects of dual-chamber pacing. *Am J Cardiol* 1984;**53**:1034–40.

26 Brignole M, Menozzi C, Lolli G, *et al.* Long-term outcome of paced and non-paced of patients with severe carotid sinus syndrome. *Am J Cardiol* 1992;**69**:1039–43.

CHAPTER 17

Structural heart disease, syncope, and risk of sudden death: selection of patients for implantable cardioverter-defibrillator therapy

Kathy L Lee, Hung-Fat Tse, Chu-Pak Lau

The only difference between syncope and sudden death is that in one you wake up

Syncope is a common presenting symptom in the community. The etiology of syncope is complex and the diagnosis is often difficult. Benign causes like neurally-mediated reflex syncope and orthostatic hypotension are common and not life threatening. However, syncope in patients with structural heart disease is associated with a worrisome prognosis and may be a predictor of sudden death. The differentiation between benign and malignant causes of syncope is for that reason an important goal of evaluation.

In the presence of organic heart disease, syncope may be caused by mechanical or electrical causes. Mechanical causes (e.g., aortic stenosis, mitral stenosis, pulmonary embolism, aortic dissection, cardiac temponade, atrial myxoma, and myocarditis) affect cardiac output and cause syncope as a result of transient hemodynamic disturbance. It is imperative to establish the diagnosis in order to correct the underlying abnormality. For electrical causes associated with an arrhythmic substrate in the ventricle, defibrillator therapy is often prescribed based on the estimated risk of sudden death (although syncope risk may persist due to the development of hypotension at the onset of the rhythm disturbance). In the presence of significant structural heart disease, implantable cardioverter-defibrillator (ICD) therapy is indicated when ventricular arrhythmia is documented, inducible by programmed electrical stimulation, or considered highly likely after extensive investigation [1–3]. Device therapy is also indicated when diagnostic work-up reveals an underlying condition that warrants implantation of defibrillator according to contemporary practice guidelines regardless of the presenting symptom of syncope. Ablation of arrhythmia substrate may

Syncope and Transient Loss of Consciousness, 1st edition. Edited by David G Benditt *et al.*
© 2007 Blackwell Publishing, ISBN: 978-1-4051-7625-5.

also be appropriate in certain cases. There is no data to support the empirical use of antiarrhythmic agents in patients with structural heart disease and syncope.

Syncope in patients with coronary artery disease

In the presence of coronary artery disease, syncope may be due to acute myocardial ischemia, ventricular tachyarrhythmias, or other causes such as bradycardia, neurally-mediated reflex syncope, and orthostatic hypotension. The work-up for patients with syncope and who are at risk of coronary artery disease should include evaluation of myocardial ischemia. If there is a history of prior myocardial infarction, cardiac electrophysiology testing is indicated for risk stratification. In patients with coronary artery disease, inducibility of ventricular tachycardia and ventricular fibrillation on electrophysiology testing correlates with a high cardiac mortality, and a negative test predicts low risk of sudden death [4]. ICD therapy improves the outcome of these patients. According to current recommendations, for patients with remote myocardial infarction, symptomatic heart failure, and left ventricular dysfunction, ICD is indicated for primary prevention of sudden death even in the absence of syncope or a positive electrophysiology testing [1]. In patients with unexplained syncope, coronary artery disease, and preserved left heart function, electrophysiology testing is useful for guidance of therapy, although the yield may be low. In the absence of inducible ventricular tachyarrhythmias, one may consider a conservative approach or proceed to use of an event monitor or an implantable loop recorder to fully clarify the problem.

Syncope in patients with nonischemic dilated cardiomyopathy

Syncope in patients with nonischemic dilated cardiomyopathy may be due to ventricular arrhythmia, bradycardia, supraventricular arrhythmia, or orthostatic hypotension. Neurally-mediated syncope is much less likely, as severe myocardial dysfunction precludes the phase of left ventricular hypercontractility in the generation of vagal response [3]. Syncope is an ominous symptom in heart failure, as both total mortality and sudden death are increased. Around 45% of patients with advanced heart failure who presented with cardiac syncope died suddenly after 1 year [5]. In addition, 70% of patients who presented with cardiac arrest or ventricular arrhythmia had at least one prior syncope spell.

There is little role for electrophysiology testing in the evaluation of syncope in nonischemic dilated cardiomyopathy. Inducibility of ventricular tachyarrhythmias is not predictive of future risk and not useful in guiding therapy. However, it may uncover certain conditions, such as sinus node dysfunction, atrioventricular (AV) conduction abnormality, and bundle branch reentry tachycardia.

The survival benefit resulting from ICD therapy in patients with nonischemic dilated cardiomyopathy and syncope has not been established in a randomized trial, but a number of studies have shown improvement in outcome. A nonrandomized study showed that patients with nonischemic dilated cardiomyopathy referred for heart transplant who received an ICD for unexplained syncope had better survival and less sudden death compared with similar patients treated by conventional medical therapy [6]. When patients with nonischemic dilated cardiomyopathy who received ICD for unexplained syncope despite a negative electrophysiology test were compared with similar patients who received the device for cardiac arrest, it was found that the rates of appropriate device shocks were similar [7]. In nonischemic dilated cardiomyopathy, increased age and depressed left ventricular ejection fraction are predictive of mortality. Recent defibrillator trials of primary prevention like the Defibrillator in Nonischemic Cardiomyopathy Treatment Evaluation (DEFINITE) [8] and Sudden Cardiac Death in Heart Failure Trial (SCD-HeFT) [9] have demonstrated the efficacy of device therapy in patients with nonischemic dilated cardiomyopathy and low ejection fraction. However, these are primary prevention trials by design, and patients with a history of syncope were excluded. In class III and IV heart failure patients with widened QRS and ejection fraction less than or equal to 35%, cardiac resynchronization therapy in combination with an ICD should be considered independent of ischemic or nonischemic etiology [1].

Syncope in other forms of structural heart disease

Certain cardiac conditions are associated with an increased risk of ventricular arrhythmia and sudden death. Unexplained syncope in these patients is usually regarded as highly suggestive of ventricular arrhythmia, and defibrillator implantation is considered reasonable. These conditions include hypertrophic cardiomyopathy and arrhythmogenic right ventricular dysplasia.

In hypertrophic cardiomyopathy, apart from common causes of syncope, left ventricular outflow obstruction, atrial arrhythmia, and myocardial ischemia may result in syncope. ICD therapy is indicated for documented ventricular arrhythmia or cardiac arrest. It is also indicated for primary prevention of sudden death in high-risk patients. Identification of other risk factors may be useful for assessment, including family history of sudden death, markedly increased left ventricular wall thickness ($\geq$30 mm during diastole), abnormal exercise hemodynamics, nonsustained ventricular tachycardia, and genetic mutation. When no other causes are identified, unexplained syncope alone is regarded as a high-risk indicator and defibrillator therapy is considered reasonable. A high rate of appropriate defibrillator discharge has been reported in high-risk patients who received the ICD for primary prevention [10]. The role of cardiac electrophysiology study is controversial in the evaluation of syncope in patients with hypertrophic cardiomyopathy.

In arrhythmogenic right ventricular dysplasia, sudden death and ventricular arrhythmia are common presenting features. A history of syncope and extensive disease with left ventricular involvement are high-risk predictors of sudden death. The role of cardiac electrophysiology study in risk stratification is controversial, and the role of genetic study is not established. Appropriate defibrillator discharge rate is high in patients who received device therapy for primary or secondary prevention of sudden death [11]. The incidence of appropriate defibrillator discharge due to ventricular tachyarrhythmias in patients presented with unexplained syncope is comparable to that in patients presented with hemodynamically significant ventricular tachycardia.

Is syncope a surrogate of sudden cardiac death?

In patient with class III and IV heart failure of both ischemic and nonischemic etiologies, the occurrence of syncope was associated with a sudden death rate of 45% in 1 year compared with 12% for those who never had syncope [5]. Furthermore, patients with syncope due to a noncardiac cause had a similar rate of sudden death (39%) when compared with those with syncope that was attributed to a cardiac cause (49%). This may be explained by the poor hemodynamic tolerance to other causes of syncope like neurocardiogenic syncope, which may induce global ischemia in patients with poor left ventricular function. These patients may also have an impaired autonomic reflex response and hence worse prognosis. Taken together, patients with advanced structural heart disease and syncope have a high risk of sudden death regardless of the cause of syncope. In addition, when treated with an ICD, they are more likely to receive appropriate device therapy than those who had defibrillators implanted purely for primary prevention. Furthermore, among patients with advanced heart failure, hypertrophic cardiomyopathy, or arrhythmogenic right ventricular dysplasia, those who received an ICD for unexplained syncope had a high rate of appropriate defibrillator shocks comparable to those who presented with documented ventricular tachyarrhythmias [7, 10, 11].

Current opinion and future directions

It is well established that inducibility at electrophysiology testing predicts occurrence of ventricular arrhythmia in the setting of coronary artery disease, and electrophysiology-guided therapy with an ICD improves outcome. In general, data support the use of defibrillators in patients with advanced heart failure and unexplained syncope [1–3]. However, it is also important to evaluate the patient carefully to exclude confounding causes. Common conditions like neurally-mediated reflex syncope and orthostatic hypotension induced by heart failure medications (i.e., vasodilators, diuretics, etc.) need to be considered. Sinus node dysfunction, conduction abnormalities, atrial arrhythmia, and proarrhythmic effects must be considered as well.

Aggressive treatment should be given for underlying myocardial ischemia or heart failure. In patients with advanced structural heart disease, when other reasons of syncope have been excluded, ICD therapy is recommended (as shown in Table 17.1) if the patient has a reasonable expectation of survival

Table 17.1 Indication of electrophysiology testing and ICD in patients with syncope, structural heart disease, and no documented ventricular arrhythmia [9–11].

Recommendation	Level of evidence*
EP testing	
Class I (general agreement of benefit of EP testing)	
In evaluation of syncope in patients with impaired LV function or structural heart disease	B
Class IIa (weight of evidence is in favor of usefulness of EP testing)	
In evaluation of syncope when bradyarrthythmias or tachyarrhythmias are suspected and in whom noninvasive diagnostic studies are not conclusive	B
Class IIb (usefulness of EP testing is less well established)	
In evaluation of syncope in patients with a high risk for life-threatening ventricular arrhythmia, such as hypertrophic cardiomyopathy and arrhythmogenic right ventricular dysplasia	C
Implantable cardioverter-defibrillator	
Class I (general agreement of benefit with ICD therapy)	
Syncope with clinically relevant and hemodynamically significant VT or VF is induced when drug therapy is not tolerated or not preferred	A
Class IIa (weight of evidence is in favor of usefulness of ICD)	
1. Unexplained syncope in patients with LV dysfunction and nonischemic dilated cardiomyopathy	C
2. Unexplained syncope in patients with certain cardiomyopathies with a high risk for life-threatening ventricular arrhythmia, such as hypertrophic cardiomyopathy and arrhythmogenic right ventricular dysplasia	C
Class IIb (usefulness of ICD is less well established)	
1. Syncope attributable to ventricular tachyarrhythmia in patients awaiting cardiac transplantation	C
2. Syncope in patients with advanced structural heart disease in which thorough investigation has failed to find out the cause	C
Class III (ICD is not effective and may be harmful)	
1. Syncope in patients with NYHA class IV drug refractory heart failure who are not candidates for cardiac transplantation	C
2. Syncope in patients who are not candidates for ICD (e.g., significant psychiatric diseases or terminal illnesses with limited life expectancy)	C

* Level of evidence: level A, data derived from multiple randomized clinical trials or meta-analysis; level B, data derived from a single randomized trial or nonrandomized studies; level C, consensus opinion of experts, case studies, or standard of care.
EP, electrophysiology study; ICD, implantable cardioverter-defibrillator; LV, left ventricular; NYHA, New York Heart Association; VF, ventricular fibrillation; VT, ventricular tachycardia.

and a good functional status. Device implantation is costly and not without inherent risk or complication; therefore, refined patient selection is desirable. Newer technology such as implantable loop recorders and microvolt T-wave alternans may improve the diagnostic yield and better stratify patients with structural heart disease and syncope.

References

1 Zipes DP, Camm AJ, Borggrefe M, *et al*. ACC/AHA/ESC 2006 guidelines for management of patients with ventricular arrhythmias and the prevention of sudden cardiac death—executive summary. *J Am Coll Cardiol* 2006;**48**:1064–108.

2 Gregoratos G, Abrams J, Epstein AE, *et al*. ACC/AHA/NASPE 2002 guideline update for implantation of cardiac pacemakers and antiarrhythmia devices: summary article. A report of the American College of Cardiology/American Heart Association Task Force on Practice Guidelines (ACC/AHA/NASPE Committee to Update the 1998 Pacemaker Guidelines). *Circulation* 2002;**106**:2145–61.

3 Strickberger SA, Benson DW, Biaggioni I, *et al*. AHA/ACCF scientific statement on the evaluation of syncope. *J Am Coll Cardiol* 2006;**47**:473–84.

4 Brembilla-Parrot B, Suty-Selton C, Beurrier D, *et al*. Difference in mechanisms and outcomes of syncope in patients with coronary disease or idiopathic left ventricular dysfunction as assessed by electrophysiologic testing. *J Am Coll Cardiol* 2004;**44**:594–601.

5 Middlekauff HR, Stevenson WG, Stevenson LW, *et al*. Syncope in advanced heart failure: high risk of sudden death regardless of origin of syncope. *J Am Coll Cardiol* 1993;**21**:110–16.

6 Fonarow GC, Feliciano Z, Boyle NG, *et al*. Improved survival in patients with nonischemic advanced heart failure and syncope treated with an implantable cardioverter-defibrillator. *Am J Cardiol* 2000;**85**:981–5.

7 Knight BP, Goyal R, Pelosi R, *et al*. Outcome of patients with non-ischemic dilated cardiomyopathy and unexplained syncope treated with an implantable defibrillator. *J Am Coll Cardiol* 1999;**33**:1964–70.

8 Kadish A, Dyer A, Daubert JP, *et al*. Prophylactic defibrillator implantation in patients with nonischemic dilated cardiomyopathy. *N Engl J Med* 2004;**350**:2151–8.

9 Bardy GH, Lee KL, Mark DB, *et al*. Amiodarone or an implantable cardioverter-defibrillator for congestive heart failure. *N Engl J Med* 2005;**352**:225–37.

10 Maron BJ, Shen WK, Link MS, *et al*. Efficacy of implantable cardioverter-defibrillators for the prevention of sudden death in patients with hypertrophic cardiomyopathy. *N Engl J Med* 2000;**342**:365–73.

11 Corrado D, Leoni L, Link MS, *et al*. Implantable cardioverter-defibrillator therapy for prevention of sudden death in patients with arrhythmogenic right ventricular cardiomyopathy/dysplasia. *Circulation* 2003;**108**:3084–91.

CHAPTER 18

Channelopathies as a cause of syncope

T Boussy, Pedro Brugada

Introduction

As described in previous chapters, syncope can be the first clinical manifestation of organic heart diseases, such as valvulopathies, hypertrophic cardiomyopathies, and congenital cardiac malformations. On the other hand, there is a wide range of primary electrical abnormalities where in the majority of cases syncope is the result of (hemodynamically compromising) ventricular arrhythmias. Here, the loss of consciousness typically has a sudden onset without prodrome and terminates spontaneously. If the arrhythmia is terminated by resuscitation, it is defined as aborted sudden arrhythmic death. In most of these cases an arrhythmogenic substrate, such as ventricular scar tissue or an accessory pathway, can be identified. In the absence of macroscopic structural heart disease, malignant arrhythmias can occur due to altered depolarization/repolarization of cardiac myocytes based on impaired ion channel function in the cardiac cell membrane. These genetically inherited "channelopathies" include the long QT syndrome, short QT syndrome, Brugada syndrome (BgS), and catecholaminergic polymorphic ventricular tachycardia.

Long QT syndrome

The long QT syndrome is characterized by prolongation of the QT interval (>500 ms) on the surface electrocardiography (ECG) and a propensity to develop torsade de pointes [1]. Over 200 mutations on seven different genes have been identified in approximately 60% of clinically diagnosed congenital long QT syndromes [2]. This genetic heterogeneity leads to different genetic subgroups with different clinical profiles (Figure 18.1):
• Long QT1 syndrome: Typically shows a long T-wave duration on the surface ECG. The trigger for cardiac arrhythmia is sympathetic hyperactivity connected with exercise or emotions. They account for sudden deaths or syncopes occurring during sports (especially swimming) and can be treated with beta blockers since inhibition of the sympathetic drive is required.

Syncope and Transient Loss of Consciousness, 1st edition. Edited by David G Benditt *et al.*
© 2007 Blackwell Publishing, ISBN: 978-1-4051-7625-5.

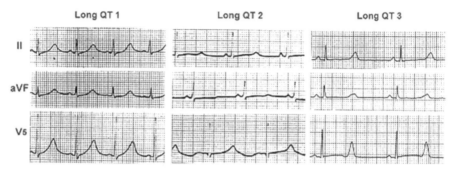

Figure 18.1 ECG recordings illustrating findings typical of LQTS 1, LQTS 2, and LQTS 3.

• Long QT2 syndrome: Characterized by small, notched T waves on the surface ECG. Emotions, rest, and acute arousal (auditory stimuli) frequently induce arrhythmic events. Sudden death or syncope in the early morning provoked by the sound of loud music or a load clock is a typical feature of long QT2 syndrome.

• Long QT3 syndrome: The surface ECG manifests a late onset of the T wave. Events occur more commonly during rest or sleep. Evidently, beta blockers are contraindicated in this group since inhibition of the sympathetic activity enhances the risk of arrhythmic events.

The acquired form of long QT syndrome consists of similar QT prolongations as in the congenital form, as a result of administration of particular drugs. These drugs practically all block the I_{kr} current (rapid potassium current), leading to impaired repolarization of the cardiac cell. Recent studies suggest that these patients are predisposed by carrying subclinical gene alterations that make them more susceptible to drug-induced QT prolongation, leading to torsade de pointes. In fact, these patients should be considered as silent carriers of the gene mutations underlying the congenital long QT syndrome.

The Brugada syndrome

In 1992, Brugada and Brugada [3] first described a new clinical entity consisting of syncopal and sudden death episodes due to malignant arrhythmias (ventricular fibrillation or polymorphic ventricular tachycardia) in the absence of structural heart disease. All patients studied showed a right-bundle-branch-like morphology with ST-segment elevation in the right precordial leads on the surface ECG. This typical ECG pattern, either occurring spontaneously or elicited by antiarrhythmic drugs, has come to be considered as a distinguishing feature of the BgS. Its prevalence varies between 0.05% (Europe and the United States) and 1% (Asia) in adult populations. In the absence of structural heart disease, BgS is responsible for at least 20% of sudden cardiac deaths.

The mean age at diagnosis is around 40 years, with a wide range between 2 months and 77 years. Males are predominantly affected (M/F ratio 3/1).

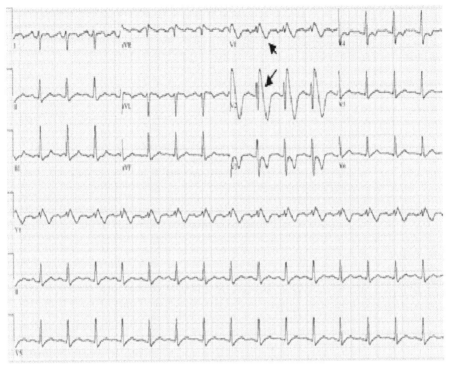

Figure 18.2 ECG findings diagnostic of Brugada syndrome (type 1 pattern, coved ST segment, BS type 1).

There is a wide spectrum of clinical manifestations, ranging from asymptomatic patients to sudden death. The majority of asymptomatic cases are family members of patients diagnosed with the syndrome who were identified during family screening. However, because of increasing awareness, sporadic asymptomatic individuals, in whom a routine ECG was recorded for various reasons, are also being increasingly recognized. Symptomatic patients present with syncopes (due to ventricular tachycardia), seizures, palpitations, nocturnal agonal respiration, or (aborted) sudden cardiac death (due to ventricular fibrillation). Up to 20% of the patients have concomitant supraventricular tachycardias, most frequently atrial fibrillation, which can also be the first presenting symptom.

Three different ECG patterns, all exhibiting ST-segment elevation in the right precordial leads, were unfortunately described [4] (Figures 18.2–18.4). Type 1 is the only pattern that is diagnostic for BgS. It consists of a coved-type ST-segment elevation ≥2 mm, followed by a negative T wave in at least one right precordial lead (V1–V3). Because of the dynamic nature of these ECG changes, with day-to-day variation in morphology and possible transient normalization, a pharmacological challenge with class I sodium channel blockers is performed to unmask the concealed coved-type ECG [5]. A definite diagnosis is made

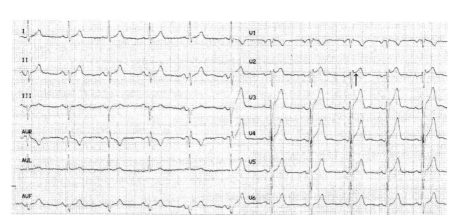

Figure 18.3 ECG findings of BS type 2 pattern suggestive of but not diagnostic of Brugada syndrome (saddleback ST segment).

when the coved-type ECG pattern, either spontaneous or drug-induced, is found in association with symptoms or documented ventricular arrhythmias or a family history of sudden cardiac death. Type 2 is a saddleback ST-segment pattern with a high initial augmentation, followed by an ST-segment elevation of ≥2 mm in at least one right precordial lead. The T wave can be positive

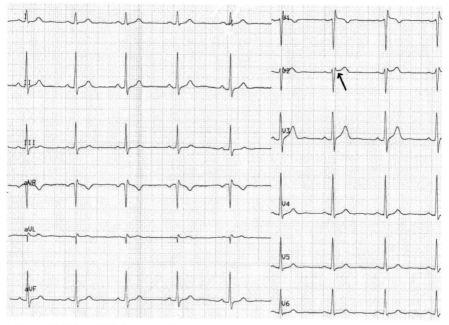

Figure 18.4 Three ECG findings of BS type 3 pattern only suggestive of Brugada syndrome (coved and saddleback ST segment).

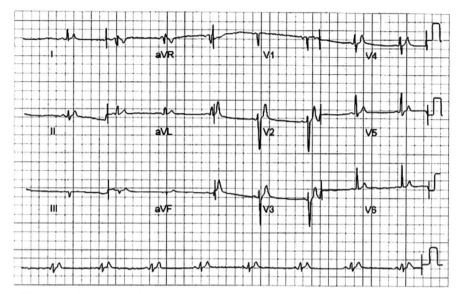

Figure 18.5 Twelve-lead ECG in a patient with short QT syndrome.

or biphasic. Type 3 ST-segment elevations are <1 mm, with either coved or saddleback morphology. It should be emphasized that the type 2 and type 3 ECG patterns are not diagnostic of BgS. In patients showing type 2 or 3 ECG pattern, BgS can be diagnosed only if conversion to the coved type I ECG occurs spontaneously or after administration of a sodium channel blocker.

The BgS is transmitted in an autosomal dominant fashion with variable expression. The first mutation linked to BgS was located in the *SCN5A* gene (chromosome 3p21) encoding for the pore-forming α subunit of the sodium channel [6]. Currently, over 70 *SCN5A* mutations have been identified accounting for approximately 25% of all BgS patients, suggesting that other gene mutations have not yet been discovered. Recently, a mutation affecting the function of the calcium channel has been described (with a doubtful association with a short QT interval).

Short QT syndrome

The short QT syndrome [7], which has been recognized as a separate clinical entity since 2003, again consists of the clinical/electrocardiographical combination of sudden death, syncope, paroxsysmal atrial fibrillation, and palpitations, with an ECG showing a shortened QT interval (<300 ms) with tall, symmetrical T waves (Figure 18.5). Because of the recent description of this disease and the lack of large population studies, there still remain a lot of questions concerning its pathophysiology. In a recent study [8], mutations resulting in an increased I_{kr} current (opposite of long QT2 syndrome) were localized in two separate genes, showing an autosomal dominant pattern of inheritance.

Catecholaminergic polymorphic ventricular tachycardia

This channelopathy should be considered in the differential diagnosis of poly-morphic ventricular tachycardia whenever episodes typically occur during exercise or emotional stress. Patients present with (aborted) sudden death or syncope, mostly during childhood [9]. The polymorphic ventricular tachycar-dia can be reproduced during an exercise test in the majority of cases.

Recent studies suggest that catecholaminergic polymorphic ventricular tachycardia is caused by an intracellular calcium overload in the cardiomy-ocyte. A similar pathophysiologic mechanism is described in digitalis intoxi-cation where electrocardiographically comparable (bidirectional) polymorphic ventricular tachycardias occur. The calcium overload results from gene muta-tions altering the function of the ryanodine receptor, which plays a crucial role in the calcium homeostasis. These mutations [10], which are transmitted as an autosomal dominant trait, seem to inhibit the intracellular Ca release in the presence of catecholamines (or sympathic activation).

Conclusion

Whenever syncope occurs, especially when characterized by a sudden onset or termination, cardiac causes need to be tracked down. However, cardiac inves-tigation should not be ceased when macroscopic or structural heart disease is excluded. The channelopathies represent a group of genetically transmittable syndromes that can easily be detected by careful and complete assessment of personal and family history and detailed inspection of the surface ECG. Misdiagnosis can lead to sudden cardiac death due to malignant ventricular arrhythmias of "unknown origin" in young and otherwise healthy individuals. If diagnosed, thorough family screening is required and the implantation of an internal defibrillator is indicated in a substantial number of patients, offering a lifelong protection against sudden cardiac death.

References

1 Schwartz PJ, Moss AJ, Vincent GM, *et al.* Diagnostic criteria for the long QT syndrome: an update. *Circulation* 1993;**88**:782–4.
2 Curran ME, Splawski I, Timothy KW, *et al.* A molecular basis for cardiac arrhythmia: HERG mutations cause long QT syndrome. *Cell* 1995;**80**:795–803.
3 Brugada P, Brugada J. Right bundle branch block, persistent ST-segment elevation and sudden cardiac death: a distinct clinical and electrocardiographic syndrome: a multicenter report. *J Am Coll Cardiol* 1992;**20**:1391–6.
4 Antzelevitch C, Brugada P, Borggrefe M, *et al.* Brugada syndrome: report of the second consensus conference. *Circulation* 2005 ;**111**:659–70.
5 Brugada R, Brugada J, Antzelevitch C, *et al.* Sodium channel blockers identify risk for sudden death in patients with ST-segment elevation and right bundle branch block but structurally normal hearts. *Circulation* 2000;**101**:510–15.
6 Chen Q, Kirsch GE, Zhang D, *et al.* Genetic basis and molecular mechanism for idiopathic ventricular fibrillation. *Nature* 1998;**392**:293–6.

7 Gaita F, Giustetto C, Bianchi F, *et al*. Short QT syndrome. A familial cause of sudden death. *Circulation* 2003;**108**:965–70.

8 Bellocq C, van Ginneken A, Bezzina CR, *et al*. Mutation in the *KCNQ1* gene leading to the short QT interval syndrome. *Circulation* 2004;**109**:2394–7.

9 Leenhardt A, Lucet V, Denjoy I, *et al*. Catecholaminergic polymorphic ventricular tachycardia in children: a 7 year follow up of 21 patients. *Circulation* 1995;**91**:1512–19.

10 Priori SG, Napolitano C, Memmi M, *et al*. Clincal and molecular characterization of patients with catecholaminergic polymorphic ventricular tachycardia. *Circulation* 2002;**106**:69–74.

CHAPTER 19

Distinguishing seizures and pseudosyncope from syncope

Adam P Fitzpatrick

In the United Kingdom, the diagnosis of epilepsy has been reported to be incorrect in up to 30% of adults and 40% of children [1–8]. Neurological sources in the United States indicate that a similar rate is prevalent there. A diagnosis of epilepsy blights life because of the impact of medication and the impact on education, employment, and childbearing.

Misdiagnoses occur partly because of confusion over terminology in patients with episodes of transient loss of consciousness (TLOC), sometimes referred to as "blackouts" (although the word "blackout" is not universally understood in this context). Often the term "syncope" is used inappropriately when "TLOC" is meant. Similarly, "seizure disorder" may be used when "epilepsy" is meant. Confusion is further compounded because seizure-like movements may occur in syncope. Indeed, anoxic seizures in syncope often mimic epileptic seizures.

Nomenclature

Commonly, inadequate appreciation of the various clinical scenarios that can cause a TLOC or apparent TLOC results in inappropriate patient care. Figure 19.1 provides a simple depiction of the relationships among collapse (an abrupt loss of postural tone), "blackouts" (TLOC), syncope (TLOC due to global impairment of cerebral perfusion), generalized epilepsy (TLOC due to asynchronous depolarization of cerebral neurones with preserved cerebral perfusion), and psychogenic "blackouts" (apparent TLOC with preserved cerebral perfusion and no evidence of asynchronous depolarization of cerebral neurones). Careful history taking can, in most cases, permit distinction among these main clinical categories and set the stage for the ultimate determination of a correct diagnosis. In this regard, from the clinical diagnostic perspective, it is important to keep in mind that syncope (which occurs in 30–50% of the population) is far more common than epilepsy (0.7–1.0% of the population). Neurally-mediated reflex syncope is by far the commonest of these conditions.

Syncope and Transient Loss of Consciousness, 1st edition. Edited by David G Benditt *et al.*
© 2007 Blackwell Publishing, ISBN: 978-1-4051-7625-5.

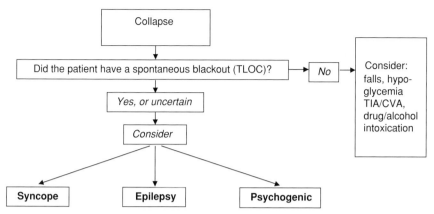

Figure 19.1 Diagram illustrating relationships among "collapse," TLOC, syncope, epilepsy, and "psychogenic pseudosyncope."

It should be noted that "falls" may occur without TLOC. This can result in a diagnostic dilemma, especially in the elderly in whom falls are often due to a failure to quickly correct for disturbances of center of gravity such as might occur when changing posture or if subjected to an inadvertent push, or even an accidental loss of footing. Aggravating factors include frailty, locomotor weaknesses, and hypotensive medications. Falls may also be due to TLOC. Unfortunately, the loss of consciousness component may be overlooked during clinical evaluation due to failure to obtain a complete history (including eyewitness accounts). A sense of suspicion must be maintained when encountering an older patient who has reportedly sustained an unexplained "fall."

In the United Kingdom, patients with TLOC are often inappropriately investigated for carotid artery disease. This is an important mistake. A transient ischemic attack causes a transient neurological deficit without loss of consciousness. TLOC is a transient loss of consciousness without neurological deficit. A carotid stenosis is *never* the cause of TLOC, unless the cerebral circulation is so compromised that the entire brain is dependent on a single vessel that in addition becomes transiently compromised.

Epilepsy, like syncope, is a clinical diagnosis. Confusion and misdiagnosis also occur because the features of "convulsive" syncope (i.e., syncope in which there is a prominent component of abnormal muscle jerking) and generalized epilepsy may appear to be very similar clinically. Both may give rise to abrupt TLOC without warning, collapse, abnormal limb movements, incontinence, and injuries.

Misdiagnosis may also stem from an overreliance on tests, when clinical evaluation and electrocardiography (ECG) are in fact far more important. Resting ECG should not be neglected in any patient with TLOC. The ECG in Figure 19.2 is from a 3-year-old female who was treated for generalized epilepsy for 2 years, without improvement, before an ECG was done and showed evidence of long QT syndrome. An implantable cardioverter-defibrillator (ICD)

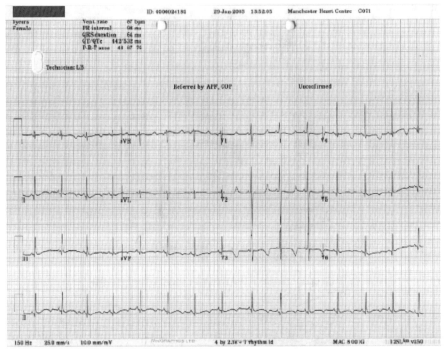

Figure 19.2 Twelve-lead electrocardiogram showing evidence of long QT in a child.

was placed and since then she had a number of ICD discharges for ventricular fibrillation.

Too much emphasis is placed on the discriminative value of tests, such as tilt-table testing and electroencephalography (EEG). Tilt-table testing is not discriminative in all comers with TLOC, where the overall yield is about 20%. An EEG is not useful for a diagnosis of epilepsy; it is used for the diagnosis of the type of epilepsy syndrome in a patient clinically diagnosed with epilepsy. An EEG is of little value in patients over 35 years.

For cardiologists, it is important to determine whether or not syncope is the cause of TLOC and whether syncope is caused by an arrhythmia. In patients with structural heart disease and syncope, there is a serious risk of death. Syncope postmyocardial infarction ventricular tachycardia has a 40–50% 1-year mortality. Similarly, patients with a primary electrical disease of the heart (long QT syndrome, Brugada syndrome, and Wolff–Parkinson–White syndrome) may be at high risk of death. However, other patients may be at low risk but still deserve a correct diagnosis and appropriate treatment. Arrhythmic syncope, where there is no structural heart disease and no primary electrical disease, cannot be diagnosed without symptom/ECG correlation, and the yield from external ECG monitoring is below 1%, *making it very cost-ineffective.*

An implantable loop recorder (ILR) should be used if symptom/ECG correlation is sought, and *this is cost-effective* and guides the effective use of permanent

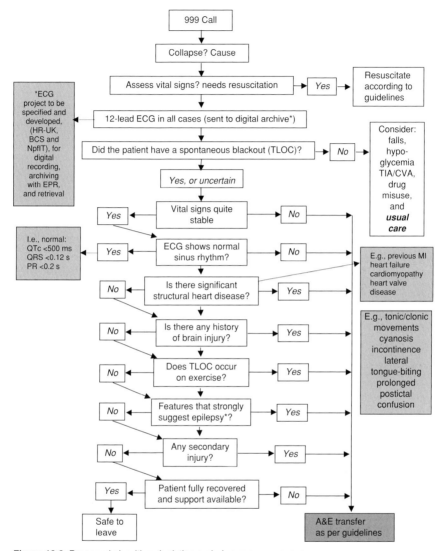

Figure 19.3 Proposed algorithm depicting ambulance crew response.

pacing in asystolic syncope. It may also make a diagnosis of convulsive asystolic syncope where generalized epilepsy has previously been diagnosed. For example, an ILR download in a 46-year-old male diagnosed with and treated for a variety of epilepsy syndromes for 20 years. After permanent pacing and withdrawal of epilepsy drugs, he has been symptom-free for 9 years revealed prolonged asystolic pauses.

The current ILR has limitations for diagnosis in TLOC patients, because it cannot provide simultaneous ECG-blood pressure-EEG/symptom correlation. Nevertheless, it can exclude or prove arrhythmic syncope in patients with

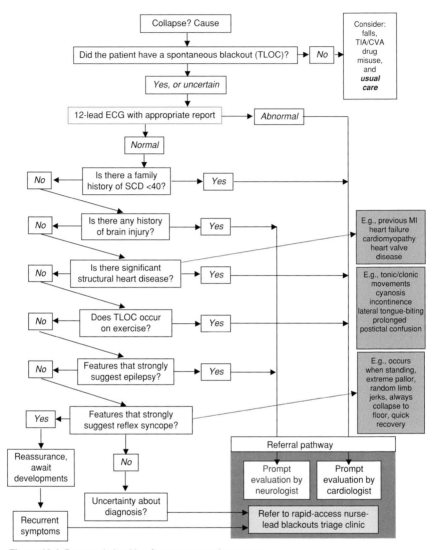

Figure 19.4 Proposed algorithm for emergency department.

normal hearts, structural heart disease, or primary electrical diseases. Future developments may permit greater versatility. However, even now the ILR is a compelling technology for assisting clinical evaluation of the cause of unexplained "collapse."

Rapid-access blackouts clinics

Given the risks and high rate of misdiagnosis of epilepsy, the need for a thorough clinical evaluation, the common features of convulsive syncope versus

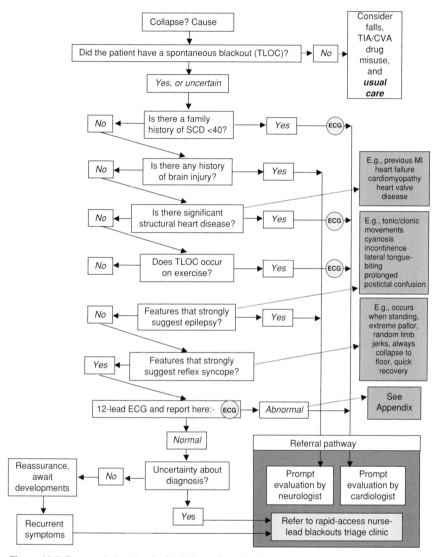

Figure 19.5 Proposed algorithm for family/attending physicians.

generalized epilepsy, and unhelpful tests, patients may suffer. Syncope management units or clinics exist, but they do not necessarily engage the multiple disciplines necessary for optimal care of patients who collapse. These disciplines include family doctors, emergency room doctors, cardiologists, neurologists, geriatricians, and increasingly other nonphysician practitioners, such as paramedics and specialist nurses.

Thus, rapid-access "blackouts" triage clinics are proposed. These clinics should be led by consultants in specialties such as cardiology, neurology,

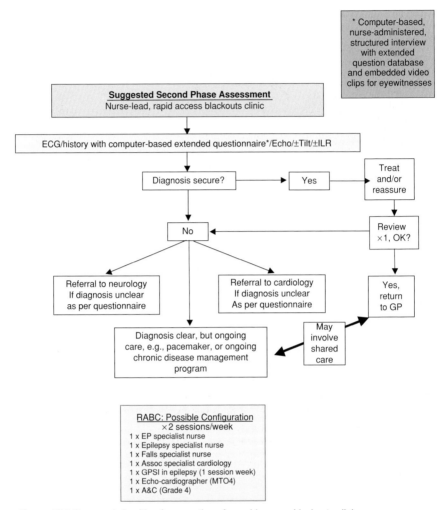

* Computer-based, nurse-administered, structured interview with extended question database and embedded video clips for eyewitnesses

Suggested Second Phase Assessment
Nurse-lead, rapid access blackouts clinic

ECG/history with computer-based extended questionnaire*/Echo/±Tilt/±ILR

Diagnosis secure?

Yes

Treat and/or reassure

No

Review ×1, OK?

Referral to neurology
If diagnosis unclear
as per questionnaire

Referral to cardiology
If diagnosis unclear
As per questionnaire

Yes, return to GP

Diagnosis clear, but ongoing
care, e.g., pacemaker, or ongoing
chronic disease management
program

May involve shared care

RABC: Possible Configuration
×2 sessions/week
1 x EP specialist nurse
1 x Epilepsy specialist nurse
1 x Falls specialist nurse
1 x Assoc specialist cardiology
1 x GPSI in epilepsy (1 session week)
1 x Echo-cardiographer (MTO4)
1 x A&C (Grade 4)

Figure 19.6 Proposed algorithm for operation of a rapid-access blackouts clinic.

and care of the elderly (geriatrics). The primary objectives of the rapid-access blackouts clinic are summarized as follows:

- develop cross-specialty experience and skills in blackouts/TLOC;
- prevent patients with TLOC being managed in disparate and often inadequately experienced settings;
- direct patients to the most appropriate specialist care promptly; and
- prevent patients becoming "stuck" in an ineffective care pathway.

In our setting, clinic care will be delivered by specialist nurses in electrophysiology, epilepsy, and falls, supervised by an appropriately experienced cardiologist. The clinical pathways recommended for ambulance crews (Figure 19.3), emergency departments (Figure 19.4), and attending physicians

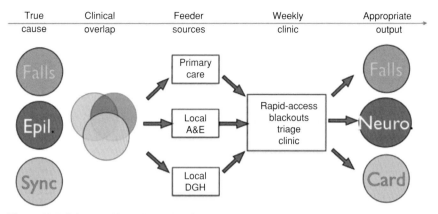

True cause	Clinical overlap	Feeder sources	Weekly clinic	Appropriate output

Figure 19.7 Schematic illustrating patient flow through a rapid-access blackouts clinic.

(Figure 19.5) are depicted. Figures 19.6 and 19.7 depict the anticipated flow pattern for patients attending such a clinic.

Summary

Misdiagnosis of seizures and syncope is a common problem with serious implications for patient well-being and quality of life. Inadequate understanding of and attention to distinctions among various conditions that can cause TLOC spells is at the core of this problem. Apart from improved physician education, the development of a structured approach to the evaluation and care of TLOC patients beginning with the initial ambulance crew to the hospital or clinic assessment is recommended. The utility of "syncope clinics" as proposed by the European Society of Cardiology Syncope Guidelines [9] may be further enhanced by the development of "rapid-access blackouts clinics" such as summarized here.

References

1 Smith D, Chadwick D. The misdiagnosis of epilepsy. *BMJ* 2002;**324**:495–6.
2 Commission on classification and terminology of the International League against Epilepsy. Proposal for a revised clinical and electroencephalographic classification of epileptic seizures. *Epilepsia* 1981;**22**:489–501.
3 Sander JWAS, Shorvon SD. Epidemiology of the epilepsies. *J Neurol Neurosurg Psychiatry* 1996;**61**:433–43.
4 Goodridge DMG, Shorvon SD. Epilepsy in a population of 6000. *BMJ* 1983;**287**:641–7.
5 Smith D, Defalla BA, Chadwick DW. The misdiagnosis of epilepsy and the management of refractory epilepsy in a specialist clinic. *Q J Med* 1999;**92**:5–23.
6 Zaidi A, Clough P, Cooper P, Scheepers B, Fitzpatrick A. Misdiagnosis of epilepsy: many seizure like attacks have a cardiovascular cause. *J Am Coll Cardiol* 2000;**36**(1):181–4.
7 Scheepers B, Clough P, Pickles C. The misdiagnosis of epilepsy: findings of a population study. *Seizure* 1998;**7**(5):403–6.

8 Stokes T, Shaw EJ, Juarez-Garcia A, Camosso-Stefinovic J, Baker R. *Clinical Guidelines and Evidence Review for the Epilepsies: Diagnosis and Management in Adults and Children in Primary and Secondary Care*. Royal College of General Practitioners, London, 2004.

9 Brignole M, Alboni P, Benditt DG, *et al.*; Task Force on Syncope, European Society of Cardiology. Guidelines on management (diagnosis and treatment) of syncope—update 2004. Executive summary. *Europace* 2004;**6**:467–537.

CHAPTER 20

Syncope and transient loss of consciousness in children and adolescents: congenital and acquired conditions

Hugh Calkins

Introduction

Syncope is a sudden transient loss of consciousness and postural tone with spontaneous recovery due to inadequate cerebral perfusion. Loss of consciousness presumably results from a reduction of blood flow to the reticular activating system located in the brainstem, and by definition it does not require electrical or chemical therapy for reversal.

The metabolism of the brain, in contrast to that of many other organs, is exquisitely dependent on perfusion, and cessation of cerebral blood flow results in loss of consciousness within approximately 10 seconds. Restoration of appropriate behavior and orientation after a syncope episode is usually immediate.

Syncope is an important clinical problem because it is common, costly, often disabling, may cause injury, and may be the only warning sign before sudden cardiac death. Although syncope occurs most commonly in adults, and increases in frequency in the very elderly, it can also occur in children. It has been estimated that up to 15% of children will experience an episode of syncope prior to the age of 18. Although the great majority of these syncope episodes will result from neurally-mediated reflex hypotension, syncope can also result from cardiac arrhythmias and/or various types of congenital or structural abnormalities of the heart. The purpose of this brief chapter is to focus on the causes of syncope in children, with a particular focus on congenital and acquired conditions.

Syncope and Transient Loss of Consciousness, 1st edition. Edited by David G Benditt *et al.*
© 2007 Blackwell Publishing, ISBN: 978-1-4051-7625-5.

Classification

The causes of transient loss of consciousness ("apparent syncope") episodes can be broken down initially into two groups: true syncope, in which the transient loss of consciousness results from cerebral hypoperfusion, and nonsyncope causes of real or apparent loss of consciousness that result from other etiologies [1, 2]. Table 20.1 shows the differential diagnosis of syncope and also these nonsyncope conditions that are indicated by an asterisk.

In pediatric patients, as in patients of any age, neurally-mediated syncope is most common. Among cardiac causes of syncope, arrhythmias are most common. The importance of considering the nonsyncope conditions when evaluating a child with apparent loss of consciousness cannot be underestimated. These "nonsyncopal" conditions (shown by an asterisk) include conditions in which consciousness is lost as a result of metabolic disorders, epilepsy, or alcohol, as well as conditions in which consciousness is only apparently lost (i.e., conversion reaction). These psychogenic causes of apparent syncope are now being recognized with increased frequency.

It is clear that patient age has an important impact on the distribution of causes of syncope. In children and young individuals, neurally-mediated syncope is by far the most common, whereas it is less so in elderly persons [3]. As compared with adults, children are less likely to experience syncope due to orthostatic hypotension, carotid sinus hypersensitivity, and some types of ventricular tachycardia (VT). This reflects the fact that many types of cardiac disease are age related and are therefore less likely to occur in children. On the other hand, neurally-mediated syncope (vasodepressor syncope) is the most common cause of syncope regardless of age. Neurally-mediated reflex syncope is covered in more detail in other sections of this book.

It is important to recognize that syncope in pediatric patients may be the first warning sign prior to death, an outcome that is devastating to the patient's family and often to their community. Some of the most worrisome causes of syncope in children are due to specific types of inherited conditions. These include long QT syncope, hypertrophic cardiomyopathy, arrhythmogenic right ventricular dysplasia (ARVD), and various types of congenital heart abnormalities [4–11].

Cardiac causes of syncope in children and adolescents

Cardiac causes of syncope, particularly tachyarrhythmias, are the second most common cause of syncope in children and adolescents. These include various types of sustained ventricular arrhythmias, and also supraventricular tachycardia (SVT). Although supraventricular tachycardia is common in children, SVTs usually result in less severe symptoms, such as palpitations, dyspnea, and light-headedness. Identification of an SVT as the cause of syncope is extremely

Table 20.1 Causes of syncope in children and adolescents.

Neurally-mediated reflex
    Carotid sinus hypersensitivity
    Vasovagal syncope
    Glossopharyngeal syncope
    Situational (cough, sneeze, swallow, micturition, and postprandial)

Orthostatic
    Autonomic insufficiency
    Idiopathic
    Volume depletion
    Drug (and alcohol) induced

Cardiac
    Anatomic
        Aortic stenosis
        Atrial myxoma
        Hypertrophic obstructive cardiomyopathy
        Coronary artery occlusion/stenosis
            Anomalous coronary (especially left)
            Coronary spasm
            Coronary artery disease (acquired)
        Kawaski syndrome
        Obstructive cardiac valvular disease
        Pericardial disease, tamponade
        Pulmonary embolus
        Pulmonary hypertension, primary or with Eisenmenger physiology
        Tetralogy of Fallot, unoperated
    Arrhythmias
        Bradyarrhythmias
            Sinus node dysfunction/bradycardia
            Atrioventricular block
            Postoperative: Mustard, Senning, Fontan, ASD, etc.
        Tachyarrhythmias
            Supraventricular arrhythmias
                Atrial tachycardia/flutter/fibrillation
                AV nodal reentrant tachycardia
                Accessory pathway mediated/WPW syndrome
        Ventricular arrhythmias
            Congenital heart disease related: Epsteins, I-transposition of the great arteries, etc.
            Inherited syndromes: long QT, hypertrophic cardiomyopathy, Brugada syndrome, arrhythmogenic right ventricular dysplasia
            Postoperative: tetralogy of Fallot, left ventricular outflow tract repair, etc.
        Malfunction of implanted pacemakers or implanted defibrillators

Vascular
    Anatomic
        Vascular steal syndromes

*Neurologic/cerebrovascular**
    "Steal syndromes"
    Arnold-Chiari malformation (uncertain role)
    Migrane (may also trigger neurally-mediated reflex syncope)
    Seizure (partial complex, temporal lobe)
    Vertebral-basilar insufficiency/transient ischemic attack

*Metabolic**
    Drugs/alcohol
    Hyperventilation (hypocapnia)
    Hypoglycemia*
    Acute hypoxemia

*Psychogenic pseudosyncope**
    Anxiety/panic disorder
    Somatization disorders

Syncope of unknown origin

*Disorders resembling syncope.

important because most types of SVTs can be cured with catheter ablation. At the present time, catheter ablation of atrioventricular (AV) nodal reentrant tachycardia, AV reentrant tachycardia, and atrial tachycardia are outpatient procedures that are associated with an efficacy of greater than 95% and a less than 1% risk of major complications. One particularly important subset of SVTs is that which occur in patients with a manifest accessory pathway and therefore carry a diagnosis of the Wolff–Parkinson–White (WPW) syndrome. Syncope may be a warning sign prior to sudden cardiac death in this patient group, and catheter ablation of the accessory pathway can be lifesaving [12, 13].

Although sustained ventricular arrhythmias are uncommon in children, reflecting the low incidence of structural cardiac abnormalities in this patient population, they can present as syncope. In the absence of structural heart disease, idiopathic VT must be considered as a potential cause of syncope. More commonly, VT causing syncope in children and adolescents occurs in the setting of acquired or congenital heart disease. Ventricular arrhythmias may also occur in patients who have undergone various types of procedures for surgical correction or palliation of congenital heart disease.

As with adults, children who have VT in the setting of structural heart disease are at increased risk for sudden death. Treatment of these arrhythmias is generally similar to the approach used in adults. Therapeutic options include antiarrhythmic drug therapy, catheter ablation, or placement of an implantable defibrillator. Because syncope is a risk factor for sudden cardiac death, careful consideration should be given to placement of an implantable cardioverter-defibrillator in patients with syncope in the setting of significant structural heart disease, and particularly when left ventricular function is impaired.

Bradyarrhythmias may also cause syncope in children and adolescents. Children can develop sick sinus syndrome or tachycardia–bradycardia syndrome. In addition, various types of cardiac surgical procedures for congenital heart disease can damage the sinus node. For example, the Mustard or Senning operation for D-transposition of the great arteries frequently damages the sinus node, perinodal structures, their blood supplies, and atrial pacemaker tissue. Although the resultant bradyarrhythmias typically present with fatigue, they may on rare occasion present with syncope.

Inherited conditions that may cause syncope in children

It is extremely important to be aware of the various types of inherited cardiac conditions that may be seen in children and may result in syncope or sudden cardiac death. These conditions often occur in the absence of any family history of syncope or sudden death. These conditions include long QT syndrome, hypertrophic cardiomyopathy, catecholaminergic polymorphic VT, the short QT syndrome, and ARVD [3–11]. Unless physicians are alert for these conditions they can be missed. All too frequently, syncope is the only warning sign prior to sudden death in a patient with a condition such as long QT syndrome, ARVD, or hypertrophic cardiomyopathy.

Diagnostic tests

Identification of the precise cause of syncope is often challenging. Because syncope usually occurs sporadically and infrequently, it is extremely difficult to either examine a patient or obtain an electrocardiogram (ECG) during an episode of syncope. For this reason, the primary goal in the evaluation of a patient with syncope is to arrive at a presumptive determination of the cause of syncope.

History and physical examination

The history and physical examination are by far the most important components of the evaluation of a patient with syncope. It is well established that the probable cause of syncope can be identified on the basis of the history and physical examination alone in more than 25% of patients [1, 12]. Maximal information can be obtained from the clinical history when it is approached in a systematic and detailed fashion. Initial evaluation should begin by determining whether the patient did, in fact, experience a syncope episode. When evaluating a patient with syncope, particular attention should then be focused on (1) determining whether the patient has a history of cardiac disease, cardiac surgery, or a family history of cardiac disease, syncope, or sudden death; (2) identifying medications that may have played a role in syncope; (3) quantifying the number and chronicity of prior syncope and presyncope episodes; (4) identifying precipitating factors including body position; and (5) quantifying the type and duration of prodromal and recovery symptoms. It is also useful to obtain careful accounts from witnesses who may have been present. The latter is particularly crucial in evaluating syncope in children, who may not be able to provide a detailed account of their symptoms.

The clinical histories obtained from patients with syncope related to AV block and VT are similar. In each case, syncope typically occurs with less than 5 seconds of warning and few, if any, prodromal and recovery symptoms. Demographic features suggesting that syncope results from an arrhythmia, such as VT or AV block, include male gender, less than three prior episodes of syncope, and increased age. Features of the clinical history that point toward a diagnosis of neurally-mediated syncope include palpitations, blurred vision, nausea, warmth, diaphoresis, or light-headedness before syncope and the presence of nausea, warmth, diaphoresis, or fatigue after syncope.

The clinical history is also valuable in distinguishing seizures from syncope. Features of the clinical history that are useful in distinguishing seizures from syncope include orientation following an event, a blue face or not becoming pale during the event, frothing at the mouth, aching muscles, feeling sleepy after the event, and a duration of unconsciousness of more than 5 minutes. Tongue biting strongly points toward a seizure rather than syncope as the cause of loss of consciousness. Other findings suggestive of a seizure as a cause of the syncope episode include (1) an aura before the episode, (2) horizontal eye deviation during the episode, (3) an elevated blood pressure and pulse during the episode, and (4) a headache following the event. Urinary or fecal incontinence can be observed in association with either a seizure or syncope but occurs more commonly in association with a seizure. Grand mal seizures are usually associated with tonic–clonic movements. It is important to note that syncope caused by cerebral ischemia can result in decorticate rigidity with clonic movements of the arms. Akinetic or petit mal seizures can be recognized by the patient's lack of responsiveness in the absence of a loss of postural tone. Temporal lobe seizures can also be confused with syncope. These seizures last several minutes and are characterized by confusion, changes in the level of consciousness, and autonomic signs such as flushing. Vertebral basilar insufficiency should be considered as the cause of syncope if syncope occurs in association with other symptoms of brainstem ischemia (i.e., diplopia, tinnitus, focal weakness or sensory loss, vertigo, or dysarthria). Migraine-mediated syncope is often associated with a throbbing unilateral headache, scintillating scotomata, and nausea.

Physical examination

After obtaining a careful history, evaluation should continue with a physical examination. In addition to a complete cardiac examination, particular attention should be focused on determining whether structural heart disease is present, defining the patient's level of hydration and detecting the presence of significant neurological abnormalities. Orthostatic vital signs are a critical component of the evaluation. The patient's blood pressure and heart rate should be obtained while he or she is supine and should then be obtained each minute for approximately 3 minutes. The two abnormalities that should be searched for are (1) early orthostatic hypotension, defined as a 20-mmHg drop in systolic blood pressure or a 10-mmHg drop in diastolic blood pressure within 3 minutes of standing, and (2) postural orthostatic tachycardia syndrome (POTS), defined as an increase of 20 beats/min or more within 5 minutes of standing with symptoms of orthostatic intolerance primarily manifest as a sense of excessively rapid heart beating upon standing. The significance of POTS in the setting of this chapter lies in its close overlap with neurally-mediated syncope [1, 13].

Laboratory and other tests

The history and physical examination are the most important components of a syncope evaluation; an ECG should also be obtained in all cases. If a cardiac cause of syncope is suspected, there should be a low threshold for obtaining an echocardiogram and/or some type of longer term arrhythmia monitoring. Other tests such as tilt-table tests, stress tests, and electrophysiology studies should be used on a case-by-case basis.

Approach to the evaluation of patients with syncope

The initial evaluation begins with a careful history, physical examination, supine and upright blood pressure, and a 12-lead ECG. Based on this initial evaluation, patients can be classified into those with true syncope and those who have not experienced true syncope. The patients with syncope can be further divided into three main groups: (1) those in whom a certain diagnosis has been established, (2) those with a suspected diagnosis, and (3) those with unexplained syncope. The subsequent use of further diagnostic testing and/or initiation of treatment can then be determined. On the basis of this initial evaluation performed in either an emergency department or an outpatient setting, the probable cause of syncope can be identified in up to 50% of patients. When this diagnostic approach has been completed, a probable cause of syncope can be determined in more than three-fourths of patients.

The European Guidelines on Management of Syncope have recently called attention to the importance of a structured care pathway in the evaluation of patients with syncope [1]. Other studies have reported favorable outcomes when a syncope evaluation unit or standardized approach to the evaluation of syncope is used.

Management of patients

The approach to treatment of a patient with syncope depends largely on the diagnosis that is established. For example, the appropriate treatment of a patient with syncope related to AV block or sick sinus syndrome would probably involve placement of a permanent pacemaker, treatment of a patient with syncope related to the WPW syndrome would probably involve catheter ablation, and treatment of a patient with syncope related to VT or in the setting of an ischemic or nonischemic cardiomyopathy would probably involve placement of an implantable defibrillator (although syncope risk may persist). For other types of syncope, optimal management may involve discontinuation of an offending pharmacological agent, an increase in salt intake, or education of the patient.

Conclusion

Transient loss of consciousness in young patients presents a higher frequency than is seen in adults of certain clinical conditions that require consideration (e.g., congenital anomalies, postsurgical corrections, and channelopathies). The evaluation strategy is similar to that recommended for adults, although greater reliance must be placed on witness (e.g., parents) accounts.

Among the more common problems faced by the physician is the appropriate restriction of physical activity and competitive sports in these patients. This must be handled on a case-by-case basis, with reference to previously published recommendations. Finally, it is important to emphasize that transient loss of consciousness in children and adolescents must always be taken seriously and be fully evaluated, as it can be a marker for occurrence of a life-threatening condition.

References

1 Brignole M, Alboni P, Benditt DG, et al. Guidelines on management (diagnosis and treatment) of syncope—update 2004. *Eur Heart J* 2004;**25**:2054–72.

2 Soteriades ES, Evans JC, Larson MG, et al. Incidence and prognosis of syncope. *N Engl J Med* 2002;**12**:878–85.

3 Strickberger SA, Benson DW, Biaggioni I, et al. AHA/ACCF Scientific Statement on the evaluation of syncope. *Circulation* 2006;**113**:316–27.

4 Priori SG, Schwartz PJ, Napolitan C, et al. Risk stratification in the long-QT syndrome. *N Engl J Med* 2003;**348**:1866–74.

5 Dalal D, Nasir K, Bomma C, et al. Arrhythmogenic right ventricular dysplasia: a United States experience. *Circulation* 2005;**25**:3823–32.

6 Antzelevitch C, Brugada P, Borggrefe M, et al. Brugada syndrome: report of the second consensus conference. *Heart Rhythm* 2005;**4**:429–40.

7 Maron BJ. Hypertrophic cardiomyopathy: a systematic review. *JAMA* 2002;**10**:1308–20.

8 Calder Kirsten K, Berbert M, Henderson SO. The mortality of untreated pulmonary embolism in emergency department patients. *Ann Emerg Med* 2005;**45**:302–10.

9 Priori SG, Napliitano C, Memmi M, et al. Clinical and molecular characterization of patients with catecholaminergic polymorphic ventricular tachycardia. *Circulation* 2002;**106**:69–74.

10 Takashi N, Shimizu W, Taguchi A, et al. Malignant entity of idiopathic ventricular fibrillation and polymorphic ventricular tachycardia initiated by premature extrasystoles origination from the right ventricular outflow tract. *J Am Coll Cardiol* 2005;**4**:1288–94.

11 Bjerregaard P, Gussak I. Short QT syndrome: mechanisms, diagnosis and treatment. *Nat Clin Pract Cardiovasc Med* 2005;**2**:84–7.

12 Friedman RA, Walsh EP, Silka MJ, et al.; North American Society of Pacing and Electrophysiology. NASPE Expert Consensus Conference: radiofrequency catheter ablation in children with and without congenital heart disease. Report of the writing committee. *Pacing Clin Electrophysiol* 2002;**25**:1000–17.

13 Blomstrom-Lundqvist C, Scheinman MM, Aliot EM, et al. ACC/AHA/ESC guidelines for the management of patients with supraventricular arrhythmias—executive summary. A report of the American College of Cardiology/American Heart Association Task Force on practice guidelines and the European Society of Cardiology Committee for practice guidelines (writing committee to develop guidelines for the management of patients with supraventricular arrhythmias) developed in collaboration with NASPE-Heart Rhythm Society. *J Am Coll Cardiol* 2003;**42**(8):1493–531.

CHAPTER 21

Transient loss of consciousness, syncope, and falls in the elderly

Rose Anne Kenny

Introduction

The incidence and prevalence of syncope increase with age due to a combination of age-related physiological and pathological changes, and age-related factors influence its consequences. These elements create diagnostic difficulties, which, in turn, have implications for subsequent investigation and management. The causes of syncope are multifactorial in this older group primarily due to increased prevalence of comorbidity, polypharmacy, and coexistence of several diagnoses. Further, the history may be unreliable and events tend to be unwitnessed, which has the potential to lead to underreporting of syncope, compounding the diagnostic dilemma.

The consequences of syncope have a greater impact on older compared with younger individuals. There is a greater risk of serious injury, in particular hip fractures (and associated increased mortality), increased rates of hospitalization, consequent loss of confidence, and reduction of independence, and a greater risk of death. Syncope in the older person poses a challenge for investigation, diagnosis, and management [1].

Falls

Syncope and falls are often considered as separate entities with different etiologies. However, an overlap between the two is increasingly evident.

A "fall" is an event in which an individual comes to rest on the ground or another level, with or without loss of consciousness. It may be categorized as "extrinsic" (where the cause is environmental) or "intrinsic" (caused by age-related or disease-related physiological and/or pathological changes). Most falls in the elderly are attributable to a combination of the two. A further classification is according to clinical characteristics. Clear recall of a slip or trip is defined as "accidental"; but if a fall and/or loss of consciousness occur *for no apparent reason*, it is considered "unexplained" or "nonaccidental" [2].

Syncope and Transient Loss of Consciousness, 1st edition. Edited by David G Benditt *et al.*
© 2007 Blackwell Publishing, ISBN: 978-1-4051-7625-5.

Clarification of a fall versus syncope must be sought, as this has prognostic implications. Such clarification relies on an accurate account of the event either from the patient or from an eyewitness. However, where a patient has cognitive impairment or dementia, the details may be inaccurate and, as episodes are unwitnessed in up to 60%, a fall or syncopal episode may go unreported [3]. The estimated annual incidence of falls in these individuals may be as high as 80%. Amnesia for loss of consciousness has been observed in cognitively normal elderly subjects who fail to recall documented falls 3 months later and in patients with carotid sinus syndrome (CSS) who present with unexplained falls and deny loss of consciousness [4]. There has also been a similar observation in young adults where syncope was induced through a sequence of hyperventilation, orthostasis, and Valsalva-like maneuver. Amnesia for loss of consciousness has been reported in postprandial hypotension and orthostatic hypotension (OH), suggesting that the phenomenon is generalized for cardiovascular syncope.

Epidemiology

Data regarding the epidemiology of syncope in the elderly are sparse. One report suggests that the incidence of syncope in persons over 70 years is at least 6% per year, with a 10% prevalence and a 30% 2-year recurrence rate. However, this is likely to be an underestimate due to the difficulties in making a diagnosis. The incidence of syncope in adults <70 years is 6.2% per 1000 person-years increasing to 11% in 70–79-year-olds and 18% in over 80-year-olds. Falls are common as persons age; at least one-third of over 65-year-olds fall once per year, half of >80-year-olds fall more than once per year, and most persons with cognitive impairment and dementia have recurrent falls.

Pathophysiology

The final common pathway for syncope is a temporary cessation of cerebral function due to sudden and transient reduction of cerebral blood flow to areas of the brain responsible for consciousness (the reticular activating system). Cerebral perfusion pressure is largely dependent on systemic arterial pressure. Any factor that decreases either cardiac output or peripheral vascular resistance diminishes systemic arterial pressure and hence cerebral perfusion. Age-related physiological and pathological changes make syncope more likely.

Age-related physiology
Baroreflex sensitivity is blunted by aging, manifesting as a reduction in heart rate response to hypotensive stimuli. Older people are prone to reduced blood volume due to excessive salt wasting by the kidneys, diminished renin-aldosterone activity, a rise in atrial natriuretic peptide, and concurrent diuretic therapy. These increase susceptibility to orthostatic hypotension (OH) and vasovagal syncope (VVS).

It is increasingly recognized that left ventricular diastolic dysfunction (with normal systolic function) is associated with aging and, indeed, may be considered part of the normal aging process. Impaired relaxation of the heart results from a series of processes, including hypertrophy, endomyocardial fibrosis, and interstitial infiltration by collagen. Changes at the cellular level of telomere length and cellular senescence underpin cardiac dysfunction.

Age-related pathology

With advancing age, many organ systems are affected by disease processes, which may be overt or covert, and this has direct and indirect implications for syncope. The most common of these processes is atherosclerosis-related disease leading to ischemic heart disease, cerebrovascular disease, and renovascular disease. Each of these may progress with age, leading to a reduction in functional reserve and development of underlying organ dysfunction. In this situation, any insult on the organ that increases demand will further compromise organ function, making it more likely to fail. This may increase the risk of syncope and the severity of the sequelae.

Left ventricular systolic dysfunction occurs most commonly secondary to ischemic heart disease. In this situation any superadded brady- or tachyarrhythmia may reduce cardiac output enough to cause syncope. Similarly, cerebrovascular disease can lead to a stepwise decline in cerebral function and cognitive impairment. Repeated transient cerebral dysfunction from recurrent hypotension and syncope may also cause cognitive impairment. Chronic renal impairment may increase the risk of syncope as a result of fluid shifts and relative intravascular volume depletion, or electrolyte disturbances with associated arrhythmias.

Essential hypertension increases in prevalence with age, which further adds to the burden of heart disease, cerebrovascular disease, and renal disease. Up to two-third of persons >70 years have hypertension. Degenerative conditions that occur due to the aging process, such as conduction tissue disease, valvular heart disease, cerebral atrophy, and locomotor disease/disability, such as osteoarthritis or Parkinson's disease, all contribute to higher age-related prevalence of syncope. In addition, several causes of syncope may coexist. The prevalence of VVS is higher in patients with carotid sinus hypersensitivity (CSH). On average, 30% of patients with CSH also have underlying sick sinus syndrome (SSS) or atrioventricular (AV) block.

Polypharmacy is increasing, with more aggressive treatment of cardiovascular disorders. It increases the risk of syncope by rendering older persons more vulnerable to hypotension and arrhythmias [5].

Common causes of syncope and falls in the elderly

The commonest causes of syncope in older adults are neurally-mediated reflex syncope (VVS and CSS), orthostatic hypotension, and cardiac arrhythmias. The prevalence of CSS increases with age and seems to parallel cardiovascular, cerebrovascular, and neurodegenerative comorbidity. Cardioinhibitory CSS has been recognized as an attributable cause of syncope in older adults in up to 20–30% of cases. Vasodepressor CSS is likely to have an equal prevalence. Up to 15% of syncope in the elderly is vasovagal. OH is an attributable cause of syncope in 20–30% of events, while cardiac arrhythmias make up 20% [6].

CSS is frequently overlooked in the elderly. It rarely occurs in adults under 50 years and increases in prevalence with advancing age. CSH is defined as a heart rate pause in excess of 3 seconds and/or a reduction in systolic blood pressure in excess of 50 mmHg during stimulation of the carotid sinus. Where syncope symptoms are attributable to these hemodynamic responses, the term CSS is applied [7]. Physiological rises in arterial blood pressure generate the stretch necessary to activate the reflex. Normally the baroreflex sensitivity declines with age, but it is enhanced in patients with CSS compared with age-matched controls.

The exact location of the pathological lesion is unknown. Although there is excessive clustering of atherosclerotic comorbidities, the abnormal response in CSS does not seem to be a purely local effect. The density of the neurodegenerative hyperphosphorylated tau protein is higher in the brainstem nuclei that regulate cardiovascular activity suggesting a central abnormality [8]. This is further supported by the high prevalence (up to 40%) of CSH in dementia with Lewy bodies (DLB) and Parkinson's disease, both of which are associated with degenerative processes in the brainstem and other features of autonomic dysfunction. Furthermore, the degree of CSM-induced hypotension correlates with the severity of cognitive impairment and the intensity of white-matter lesions in cognitive impairment that has not progressed to dementia. Whether early detection of CSH and intervention might influence long-term outcome in patients with cognitive impairment and dementia remains to be established [9, 10].

It is important to be aware of CSH as a possible attributable cause of nonaccidental falls. The prevalence of cardioinhibitory CSS in unexplained falls is high. In the SAFE PACE study, permanent pacing was applied to a group of patients with cardioinhibitory CSS. Paced patients were significantly less likely to fall than controls, and syncopal events were reduced, as were injurious events, by 70%, indicating that there is a strong association between unexplained falls and cardioinhibitory CSS [11].

In an unselected sample of older patients presenting to an accident and emergency department with unexplained or recurrent falls, VVS was present in 16–18%. Syncope results from hypotension due to vasodilatation, with varying degrees of bradycardia and/or asystole, and consequent cerebral hypoperfusion. Older patients are more likely to exhibit dysautonomic responses to head-up tilt.

OH is a reduction in systolic blood pressure of at least 20 mmHg or diastolic blood pressure of at least 10 mmHg within 3 minutes of standing. The reported prevalence of OH varies between 4 and 33% among community-dwelling elderly and makes up 14% of all diagnosed causes of syncope [12].

The prevalence and magnitude of reductions in systolic blood pressure increase with age and are associated with general frailty and excessive mortality. Similar to VVS, OH results from the breakdown of a normal reflex on standing. This is at the level of the carotid and aortic arch arterial baroreflex. Several pathological conditions are associated with OH. Common causes of OH are medications, autonomic failure, volume depletion, multiple system atrophy, and Parkinson's disease. A number of nonneurogenic conditions are also associated with or exacerbate preexisting OH. They include hemorrhage, diarrhea, vomiting, burns, hemodialysis, diabetes insipidus, adrenal insufficiency, fever, and extensive varicose veins.

With aging there is a greater coincidence of hypertension with OH. Hypertension impairs baroreflex sensitivity and restricts ventricular filling and, paradoxically, increases the risk of episodic hypotension. Hypertension may also alter the thresholds at which cerebral autoregulation occurs. As a consequence, older subjects with hypertension and orthostatic hypotension are less able to compensate and are therefore exposed to the risks of episodic cerebral ischemia and syncope [13].

With primary autonomic failure, there are three main clinical entities: pure autonomic failure, multiple system atrophy, and autonomic failure associated with idiopathic Parkinson's disease. Pure autonomic failure is a relatively benign condition previously known as idiopathic OH. It presents as orthostatic hypotension, defective sweating, impotence, and bowel disturbance but with no other neurological defects. Multiple system atrophy is associated with the poorest prognosis. Clinical features include dysautonomia and motor disturbances due to striatonigral degeneration, cerebellar atrophy, or pyramidal lesions. OH associated with Parkinson's disease can be caused by factors other than dysautonomia, such as medication side effects.

Secondary autonomic failure is most commonly due to diabetes or chronic renal failure. In the absence of well-recognized conditions causing primary or secondary autonomic failure, aging per se can be a cause of OH.

Arrhythmias cause approximately 20% of syncope episodes in older adults. Brady- and tachyarrhythmias can cause a sudden decrease in cardiac output. Bradycardias are initially compensated for by prolonged ventricular filling, resulting in increased stroke volume and maintained cardiac output. As the heart rate slows, this compensatory mechanism is overwhelmed, cardiac output falls, and syncope occurs. Similarly, mild to moderately fast tachycardias increase cardiac output but even faster heart rates result in decreased ventricular diastolic filling, reduced cardiac output, and potential syncope. Additional mechanisms in supraventricular tachycardias activate cardiac mechanoreceptors and induce neurally-mediated reflex syncope (rapid, vigorous ventricular contraction in the setting of a relatively empty ventricle). Physiological impairments associated with aging, the effects of multiple medications, and comorbidity further predispose older adults to syncope even in the setting of brief arrhythmias.

Conduction tissue disease (primarily SSS and AV node disease) and ventricular tachycardia are common arrhythmic causes of syncope in aging and are diagnosed and managed in the same manner as in younger adults.

Consequences of syncope

The impact of the consequences of syncope is substantial in the elderly due to the incidence of falls and injurious events, the prevalence of comorbid disease (such as osteoporosis), and reduced organ reserve. Certain causes of syncope are directly associated with higher mortality, such as heart block, ventricular tachyarrhythmia, and acute myocardial infarction.

Hip fractures represent one of the most important consequences of falls in the older adult and are associated with a high mortality rate. Approximately half of previously independent older patients become partly dependent and one-third become totally dependent after hip fracture. In one series, the 1-year survival was 55%. Several studies have shown symptomatic older persons with CSH to be at a particularly high risk of serious injury. Where CSH was the attributable cause of syncope or falls, 25% of patients sustained a fracture, and in another study, over 30% of persons who had unexplained falls due to CSH had a previous fracture. One case-controlled series showed reproducible CSH in 36% of patients with fractured neck of femur, compared with none from elective surgery, and 17% of outpatients. In addition to physical injury, falls can have important psychological and social consequences. Recurrent falls are one of the most common reasons cited for admission of previously independent elderly people to institutional care. Fear of falling and the postfall anxiety syndrome are also well recognized as negative consequences of falls. Loss of confidence can result in self-imposed functional limitations and dependence. The negative impact of falls on quality of life, mood, and functional capacity is even more apparent for subjects who experience unexplained recurrent falls than for those who have accidental falls.

Clinical features in older patients

Syncope may present in many ways. The key to making any diagnosis is an accurate account of the presentation, either from the patient or from an eyewitness. In older persons, the reliability and accuracy of this account may be questionable. This is primarily due to the increased incidence of cognitive impairment. However, even in cognitively normal individuals, there is a greater incidence of retrograde amnesia in which patients deny loss of consciousness, presumably due to memory loss that may be the result of the syncopal episode. In addition, many presentations of syncope are unwitnessed. As already discussed, older persons may report a fall rather than syncope, adding to the potential underdiagnosis of syncope. Furthermore, with the greater incidence of comorbidity in older adults, physicians must be cautious in attributing a cause.

Individuals who describe syncope usually also experience presyncope. However, in CSS, the symptoms are generally sudden and unpredictable and precipitated either by mechanical stimulation of the carotid sinus, such as by head turning, tight neckwear, shaving, and neck pathology, or by vagal stimuli. Head movement provokes syncope in 47% and vagal-type stimulants provoke syncope in 73%. In VVS, precipitants can be prolonged standing (or sitting), hot environments, cough, micturition, deglutition, defecation, or commonly medications. However, unlike CSS, there is usually a prodromal phase where patients feel light-headed, hot, or nauseous.

The classical history of OH is posture-induced dizziness or collapse within minutes of rising from a sitting or lying position. Symptoms are generally worse in the morning. A coat-hanger distribution of pain across the neck and shoulders often accompanies OH. Quick symptom relief occurs when the patient sits or lies supine.

The physical examination is as for younger adults but includes an evaluation of mental state, the consequences of injury, and an assessment of falls risk. Older patients have a high prevalence of cardiac disease. Consequently, careful cardiac and peripheral vascular examination should be undertaken in older syncope patients.

Assessment of the neurological and locomotor systems, including observation of gait and standing balance, should be part of the initial evaluation in older patients. Signs of Parkinson's disease and arthritic processes should be elicited.

If cognitive impairment is suspected, this should be formally evaluated with the Mini Mental State Examination (MMSE), which is a 30-item, internationally validated tool.

Investigations

Syncope and falls are intermittent, transient symptoms that cluster. Typically, patients are asymptomatic at the time of assessment, and the opportunity to capture a spontaneous event during diagnostic testing is rare. The most important elements in the evaluation of syncope in older adults are to establish whether the patient has actually experienced syncope and to select the appropriate cardiovascular investigations to define the cause. In order to attribute a diagnosis with certainty, patients must have symptom reproduction during investigation and preferably alleviation of symptoms with specific intervention during follow-up. In cognitively normal older patients with syncope or unexplained falls, the diagnostic work-up is largely the same as for younger adults but should include CSM.

CSM should be performed with continuous surface electrocardiograph (ECG) and phasic blood pressure monitoring, using digital photoplethysmography. (The blood pressure nadir in response to CSM occurs around 18 s and returns to baseline at 30 s.) In up to a third of older patients with CSS, a positive response is present only when performed in the upright position. The sensitivity of the response to CSM is increased by 51% and the diagnosis enhanced by 38% when CSM is performed in the upright position. However, care should be taken in interpretation, as CSM is a crude and unquantifiable technique that is prone to both intra- and interoperator variation. Furthermore, the prevalence of CSH is high (over 30%) in asymptomatic elderly and thus the importance of care when attributing a causal association. Seventy percent of hypersensitive responses are represented by sinoatrial arrest and AV block, and the remainder are represented by sinoatrial arrest alone. As the pattern of response is not always consistent, dual-chamber pacing is mandatory for treating the cardioinhibitory or mixed type.

Conditions where head-up tilt-table testing is warranted are evaluation of older adults with recurrent unexplained falls, evaluation of recurrent syncope, or a single syncopal event in a high-risk patient where syncope has resulted in injury or determination of cause has significant occupational consequences, and further evaluation of patients in whom an apparent cause has been established (e.g., asystole or AV block) but in whom demonstration of susceptibility to neurally-mediated reflex syncope could alter treatment choice. Relative contraindications include proximal coronary stenosis, critical mitral stenosis, clinically severe left ventricular outflow obstruction, and severe cerebrovascular disease. False-positive head-up tilt is less common in the elderly.

OH is not always reproducible in older adults. This is particularly so for drug-related or age-related OH. Diagnosis of OH involves demonstration of a postural fall in blood pressure after standing (active stand). Reproducibility of OH depends on the time of measurement and on autonomic function. The measurement should be carried out as early in the morning as is practical after maintaining a supine posture for at least 10 minutes. Phasic blood pressure measurements are more sensitive than sphygmomanometer measurements.

Autonomic function tests measure sympathetic and parasympathetic outflow using a series of maneuvers, usually a minimum of four. They include the active-stand test, deep breathing, the Valsalva-like maneuver, and cold pressor effect of placing a hand in cold water. Heart rate response tests (e.g., Valsalva maneuver, and Carotid sinus massage, among others) predominantly assess parasympathetic autonomic status, while blood pressure tests (e.g., nitroglycerine, upright tilt) principally assess the sympathetic arm of autonomic control.

Twenty-four-hour ambulatory blood pressure recordings may be helpful if medication-induced or postprandial hypotension is suspected. In older patients with OH, diurnal patterns of blood pressure are the mirror image of normal blood pressure behavior, being highest at night and lowest in the mornings (and possibly after meals). Knowledge of diurnal blood pressure behavior can guide treatment and may be particularly helpful in modifying the timing of medications.

The ECG is abnormal in up to 50% of patients presenting with syncope. However, in only 5% of these patients can a cause of syncope be determined from the ECG abnormality, which might be an arrhythmia directly associated with syncope or more commonly an abnormality that may predispose to the arrhythmia. An abnormality of the baseline ECG is an independent predictor of cardiac syncope and is associated with increased mortality. Equally, a normal ECG is associated with a low risk of cardiac syncope.

Patient-activated external loop has limitations for older patients, as activation requires manual dexterity and intact cognitive function. Implantable loop recorders are now increasingly used for older patients [14]. The clinical usefulness and cost-effectiveness of the device requires further definition particularly in the case of unexplained falls.

Treatment

Treatment should be directed toward the specific cause of syncope and to risk reduction. There are few outcome data for many of the therapies, but most strategies aim to target the purported mechanism of the condition and are the same as for younger patients. Withdrawal of culprit medications is a more frequently recommended intervention in the elderly. Vasodepressor CSH may respond to midodrine, an alpha agonist [15]. Treatment of cardioinhibitory CSS includes withdrawal of culprit medications (particularly beta blockers). In patients who have idiopathic positive CSM with symptom reproduction and a suggestive history, a permanent dual-chamber pacemaker with *rate-drop* feature is indicated.

Conclusion

In conclusion, diagnosis can be difficult due to confounding factors and more than one possible attributable cause; histories may be inaccurate or unreliable, and the situation is often complicated by comorbidity and polypharmacy. In making a diagnosis, age-related physiological and pathological processes should be considered in the context of the history and examination. Appropriate investigation can then be directed accordingly, bearing in mind the evidence base, for these tests may be more applicable to younger persons.

Similarly, in considering any treatment for syncope, evidence in the form of randomized controlled trials should be followed where possible. However, in certain areas, there are few data on interventions in the older population, particularly in the very old. In practical terms, the evidence base must therefore be extrapolated. In all patients an evaluation of risk versus benefit and a degree of pragmatism should be adopted in the absence of evidence.

References

1 Nath S, Kenny RA. Syncope in the older person: a review. *Rev Clin Gerontol* 2006;**16**:1–17.
2 O'Loughlin JL, Robitaille Y, Boivin JF, Suissa S. Incidence of and risk factors for falls and injurious falls among the community-dwelling elderly. *Am J Epidemiol* 1993;**137**:342–54.

3 Cummings SR, Nevitt MC, Kidd S. Forgetting falls: the limited accuracy of recall of falls in the elderly. *J Am Geriatr Soc* 1988;**36**:613–16.

4 Parry SW, Steen IN, Baptist M, Kenny RA. Amnesia for loss of consciousness in carotid sinus syndrome: implications for presentation with falls. *J Am Coll Cardiol* 2005;**45**:1840–3.

5 Kaufman DW, Kelly JP, Rosenberg L, Anderson TE, Mitchell AA. Recent patterns of medication use in the ambulatory adult population of the United States: the Slone Survey. *JAMA* 2002;**287**:337–44.

6 McIntosh SJ, da Costa D, Kenny RA. Outcome of an integrated approach to the investigation of dizziness, falls and syncope in the elderly referred to a syncope clinic. *Age Ageing* 1993;**22**:53–8.

7 Brignole M, Alboni P, Benditt DG, *et al.*; Task Force on Syncope, European Society of Cardiology. Guidelines on management (diagnosis and treatment) of syncope—update 2004. Executive summary. *Eur Heart J* 2004;**25**:2054–72.

8 Miller VM, Kalaria RN, Hall R, Oakley AE, Kenny RA. Medullary microvessel degeneration in multiple system atrophy. *Neurobiol Dis* 2007 [Epub ahead of print]. PMID: 17466525.

9 Kenny RA, Shaw FE, O'Brien JT, *et al.* Carotid sinus syndrome is common in dementia with Lewy bodies and correlates with deep white-matter lesions. *J Neurol Neurosurg Psychiatry* 2004;**75**(7):966–71.

10 Kenny RA, Kalaria R, Ballard C. Neurocardiovascular instability in cognitive impairment and dementia. *Ann N Y Acad Sci* 2002;**977**:183–95.

11 Kenny RA, Richardson DA, Steen N, Bexton RS, Shaw FE, Bond J. Carotid sinus syndrome: a modifiable risk factor for non-accidental falls in older adults (SAFE PACE). *J Am Coll Cardiol* 2001;**38**:1491–7.

12 Kerr SRJ, Pearse M, Brayne C, Davis R, Kenny RA. CSH in asymptomatic older persons. *Arch Intern Med* 2006;**5**:166–8.

13 Parry SW, Steen N, Baptist M, Fiaschi KA, Parry O, Kenny RA. Cerebral autoregulation is impaired in CICSS. *Heart* 2006;**92**:792–7.

14 Farwell DJ, Freemantle N, Sulke AN. Use of implantable loop recorders in the diagnosis and management of syncope. *Eur Heart J* 2004;**25**:1257–63.

15 Moore A, Watts M, Sheehy T, Lyons D. Treatment of vasodepressor carotid sinus syndrome with midodrine: a randomized control pilot study. *J Am Geriatr Soc* 2005;**53**:114–18.

CHAPTER 22

Drug-induced (iatrogenic) syncope

Gerald V Naccarelli

Prescribed drugs are a common iatrogenic cause of near syncope and syncope [1–6]. Drug-induced syncope is more common in the elderly, who have age-related impaired baroreceptor reflex mechanisms, decreased arterial compliance in addition to an impaired beta-receptor sensitivity, and renin–angiotensin system [7]. One study of 822 patients reported that causes of syncope in 6.8% of the patients were medication related, although the overall incidence was not different between cardiac and noncardiac patients [8].

In screening for this cause of syncope, a complete drug history should include ascertaining if there is a time correlation between symptoms (near syncope and syncope) and recent dose changes, the addition of new drugs, or the use of over-the-counter remedies [3]. Recent-onset syncope in a patient who has been on a drug that can cause hypotension for years should lead to a search for another cause. Autonomic dysfunction and/or hypovolemia (e.g., dehydration) can aggravate or be part of the hemodynamic issue in patients with drug-induced syncope. In patients who have become hypovolemic from vomiting, diarrhea, gastrointestinal bleeding, fever, or decreased oral intake, there is no extra reservoir of blood in the venous system to compensate for gravitational pooling of blood upon standing. Demonstration of significant orthostatic hypotension on physical examination is usually possible if the patient is assessed carefully near the time of the episode. However, this is often not the case, and it is often necessary to make the diagnosis by inference based on a careful history taking.

Causes of drug-induced syncope

Table 22.1 gives drugs that are among the ones most associated with causing drug-induced syncope or near syncope [4]. As has been noted above, the diagnosis of drug-induced syncope can be made if there is a temporal relationship with the start of a drug or change in dose and the new onset of symptoms and if the syncope is ameliorated once the offending agents is discontinued. (This latter point of course may only be convincingly determined by prolonged follow-up.) In this situation any further evaluation is not indicated. If symptoms do

Syncope and Transient Loss of Consciousness, 1st edition. Edited by David G Benditt *et al.*
© 2007 Blackwell Publishing, ISBN: 978-1-4051-7625-5.

Table 22.1 Drugs that can cause orthostatic hypotension, near syncope, and syncope.

Alpha blockers
Beta blockers
Bromocriptine
Diuretics
Insulin
Monoamine oxidase inhibitors
Narcotics
Sedatives
Nitrates
Phenothiazines
Sildenafil
Sympatholytics
Sympathomimetics
Tricyclic antidepressants
Vasodilators
Vincristine
Alcohol

not improve on withdrawing the potential offending agent and after rendering the patient euvolemic, one should search further for an alternative explanation for the patient's symptoms.

In the elderly population, the adverse effects of multiple medications, especially antihypertensive and antidepressant drugs, are common causes of drug-induced syncope (estimated at approximately 5% of all causes of syncope in older patients [9]). In the cardiac population, nitrates, diuretics, beta blockers, and vasodilators are common offending agents. In an elderly male population, alpha blockers used to treat benign prostatic hypertrophy are a common offender especially if patients are already on other vasodilating agents. Alpha blockers, mixed alpha- and beta-blocking drugs, such as labetalol, or other vasodilating drugs, such as hydralazine, cause more orthostatic hypotension than a pure beta blocker. Quinidine can cause vasodilation and hypotension secondary to the drug's alpha-antagonistic effects. Calcium-channel blockers, such as nifedipine, are more likely to cause orthostatic hypotension than verapamil and diltiazem due to their more pronounced peripheral vasodilating effects. In patients with systolic dysfunction, the combination of a decreased ejection fraction along with multiple drugs (beta blockers, angiotensin-converting enzyme inhibitors, and diuretics) can often cause hypotension and syncope. The increasing use of sildenafil and other drugs for male sexual dysfunction has added new offending agents in such patients. The combination of phosphodiesterase inhibitors and nitrates should be avoided.

In some patients, syncope may be drug induced secondary to a proarrhythmia [10]. Beta blockers, amiodarone, verapamil, and diltiazem can slow heart rate enough to cause hemodynamic symptoms. Tricyclic antidepressants, sotalol, quinidine, dofetilide, as well as many other drugs can cause

Table 22.2 Partial list of drugs prolonging the QT interval and causing torsade de pointes.

Ajmaline	Levofloxacin
Amantadine	Lithium
Amiodarone	Mesoridazine
Amitriptyline	Methadone
Bepridil	Methylphenidate
Clarithromycin	Moxifloxacin
Chloroquine	Nortriptyline
Chlorpromazine	Paroxetine
Desipramine	Pentamidine
Disopyramide	Procainamide
Dofetilide	Quinidine
Doxepin	Risperidone
Droperidol	Sertraline
Erythromycin	Sotalol
Haloperidol	Thioridazine
Ibutilide	Venlafaxine
Imipramine	Ziprasidone
Ketoconazole	

QT prolongation and torsade de pointes, which may be more likely to occur if the patient has low potassium or magnesium levels (Table 22.2).

Prognosis

The prognosis of patients with drug-induced syncope appears to be benign and probably best predicted by comorbid conditions. In one study [8], patients with drug-induced syncope, including a subgroup with vasovagal syncope, had mortality rates similar to those without syncope and better than those with syncope of unknown cause or neurologic or cardiac syncope. On the other hand, physical injury is an important concern especially in the elderly. For instance, in a group of older fainters of various etiologies of which drug induced was only a portion, Ungar *et al.* reported an approximate 10% incidence of fractures related to faints and "falls" [9].

Treatment

If it is established that the syncope is drug induced, the clinician has to determine the safety of withdrawing the medication. If the drug can be safely discontinued, one needs to observe for clinical improvement in orthostatic hypotension and symptoms. If the drug cannot be completely stopped, then a dose reduction may be beneficial. In this case, intravenous fluids, increasing oral intake of fluids, or the use of added salt in the diet, fludrocortisone, midodrine, and/or support hose may all be beneficial (but possibly a problem if the patient is in part being treated for hypertension or heart failure). If the patient is severely anemic, transfusion with packed red blood cells can correct the situation.

In patients who have syncope secondary to drug-induced bradyarrhythmia, treatment includes either withdrawing the offending agent, decreasing the dose, or inserting a permanent pacemaker. In the setting of drug-induced torsade de pointes, treatment includes withdrawal of the offending agents, correcting hypokalemia or hypomagnesemia, and avoiding any drugs that can prolong action potential duration [9]. Overdrive pacing to prevent pause-dependent ventricular tachycardia can also be used when necessary.

Conclusion

Drug-induced syncope is a frequent problem, and a particularly critical issue in older individuals who tend to be taking more medications and who at the same time are at increased risk of fainting. A careful history taking is essential to make the diagnosis. However, treatment can be difficult, as the medications at "fault" are often being used to manage important comorbidities.

References

1 Lipsitz LA. Orthostatic hypotension in the elderly. *N Engl J Med* 1989;**321**:952–7.

2 Hanlon JT, Linzer M, MacMillan JP, Lewis IK, Felder AA. Syncope and presyncope associated with probable adverse drug reactions. *Arch Intern Med* 1990;**150**:2309–12.

3 Linzer M, Yang EH, Estes NAM, Wang P, Vorperian VR, Kapoor WN. Diagnosing syncope. Part 1: Value of history, physical examination, and electrocardiography. The clinical efficacy assessment project of the American College of Physicians. *Ann Intern Med* 1997;**126**:989–96.

4 Campbell AJ. Drug treatment as a cause of falls in old age: a review of offending agents. *Drugs Aging* 1991;**1**:289–302.

5 Brignole M, Alboni P, Benditt DG, *et al.*; Task Force on Syncope, European Society of Cardiology. Guidelines on management (diagnosis and treatment) of syncope. Executive summary. *Europace* 2004;**6**:467–537.

6 Strickberger SA, Benson WA, Biaggioni I, *et al.* AHA/ACCF scientific statement on the evaluation of syncope. *Circulation* 2006;**113**:316–27.

7 Grubb BP, Karas B. Clinical disorders of the autonomic nervous system associated with orthostatic intolerance: an overview of classification, clinical evaluation and management. *Pacing Clin Electrophysiol* 1999;**22**:798–810.

8 Soteriades ES, Evans JC, Larson MG, *et al.* Incidence and prognosis of syncope. *N Engl J Med* 2002;**347**:878–85.

9 Ungar A, Mussi C, Del Rossi A, *et al.* Diagnosis and characteristics of syncope in older patients referred to geriatrics departments. *J Am Geriatr Soc* 2006;**54**:1531–6.

10 Naccarelli GV, Wolbrette DL, Luck JC. Proarrhythmia. *Med Clin North Am* 2001;**85**:503–27.

PART 4

Economic and research aspects

Syncope and the competitive athlete: recommendations for evaluation and permission to compete

Franco Giada, Antonio Raviele

Syncope is a common medical issue in the general population. Syncopal spells may also occur in well-conditioned athletes at rest, as well as during training or competition, leading to anxiety among relatives, coaches, and the athletes themselves. Although population studies are scarce, syncope seems to be particularly frequent in highly trained endurance athletes [1].

Evaluation of athletes with syncope

Most athletes with transient loss of consciousness show no evidence of cardiovascular disease (CVD). These individuals are usually affected by benign neurally-mediated syncope (NMS). However, syncope may also be the first manifestation of severe CVD, and as such it may be a harbinger of sudden death. Moreover, the occurrence of syncope in athletes, especially in those engaged in certain risky activities (climbing, car racing, etc.), is associated with a major risk of physical injuries. Finally, when syncopal spells are recurrent, they can become a significant disability for the athlete and a concern for the team. Thus, although in a general population a negative complete evaluation may be reassuring, this is not necessarily true for athletes: the failure to establish a diagnosis may lead to continued uncertainty and often precludes these athletes from resuming sports activity.

Evaluation of athletes with syncope does not differ significantly from that recommended by European Society of Cardiology guidelines in general population. However, because of the quite low specificity of reflexivity maneuvers (e.g., tilt-table testing and carotid sinus massage) in athletes (see below), and since the crux of the issue is to separate individuals with a normal heart from those with CVD, the initial evaluation should also include (besides medical history, physical examination, and a closely scrutinized electrocardiogram (ECG)) an echocardiogram (ECHO) [2, 3] (Figure 23.1).

Syncope and Transient Loss of Consciousness, 1st edition. Edited by David G Benditt *et al.*
© 2007 Blackwell Publishing, ISBN: 978-1-4051-7625-5.

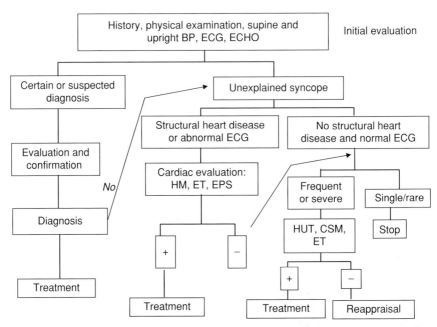

Figure 23.1 Strategy for evaluating the athlete with syncope. The figure shows the diagnostic flow chart of athletes with syncope. BP, blood pressure; ECG, electrocardiogram; ECHO, echocardiogram; ET, exercise test; HM, Holter monitoring; EPS, electrophysiologic study; HUT, head-up tilt testing; CSM, carotid sinus massage. (Modified by ESC guidelines on management of syncope. *Eur Heart J*, 2004.)

A thorough description of the syncopal episode should be obtained in all syncope patients but in particular the competitive athlete. In addition, a detailed review of any cardiac conditions, dietary habits, and current therapeutic or recreational drugs is essential. It is also necessary to ascertain the types and the degree of training the athlete is engaged in, to interpret the results of ECG and ECHO and to develop a differential diagnosis between "athlete's heart" and some pathological conditions [4, 5]. In many cases, the initial evaluation is enough to lead to a certain or suspected diagnosis.

Head-up tilt testing

When the initial evaluation has excluded the presence of CVD, head-up tilt testing (HUT) may be employed to assess the neurally-mediated origin of syncope. However, it must be underlined that the real diagnostic value of HUT in athletes is still not completely known. When data collected from athletes are compared with those of the general population of the same age, the sensitivity of HUT seems higher (Table 23.1) and the specificity lower (Table 23.2), especially in endurance athletes [1, 6–8]. This low specificity, explained by a decreased orthostatic tolerance related to the training-induced adaptations on

Table 23.1 Positive rate of tilt-table testing in athletes with syncope.

Author	No. of athletes	Gender	Age (yr)	Sport	Positive rate
Grubb (1993)	24	12 M	18 ± 3	Mixed	19/24 (79%)
Sakaguchi (1995)	10	6 M	21 ± 5	Mixed	9/19 (90%)
Calkins (1995)	17	8 M	28 ± 17	Mixed	17/17 (100%)
Sneddon (1994)	5	3 M	42 ± 15	NA	5/5 (100%)
Osswald (1994)	3	3 M	22–35	Mixed	3/3 (100%)
Manari (1996)	6	5 M	30 ± 5	Endurance	5/6 (83%)
Tortorella (1998)	7	7 M	35 ± 3	Endurance	6/7 (86%)
Colivicchi (2002)	33	13 M	$21 + 3$	Mixed	22/33 (67%)

cardiovascular and autonomic nervous systems, requires cautious interpretation of the results.

Exercise testing
Exercise testing (ET) is always indicated when there is a presence or suspicion of CVD, and in exercise-related syncope. However, ET has demonstrated, even when employing a modified protocol with abrupt termination, a quite low sensitivity in the evaluation of exercise-induced NMS [1, 7, 8].

Electrophysiologic study
Electrophysiologic study (EPS) is indicated in the presence of CVD. EPS could also be considered in athletes with unexplained syncope and without CVD in the following situations: syncope preceded by palpitations, syncope occurring without warning symptoms and/or in supine position, professional athletes, athletes who wish to participate in potentially traumatic sports, and subjects with family history of sudden death. However, EPS in athletes without CVD has shown a very low diagnostic value [7–10].

Implantable loop recorder
In athletes with recurrent syncope and negative diagnostic evaluation, a long-term ECG monitoring by means of implantable loop recorder (ILR) must be considered [2, 4]. Although this strategy implicitly requires waiting for another syncope event, it has the merit of providing as definitive a diagnosis as is

Table 23.2 Positive rate of tilt-table testing in athletes without syncope.

Author	No. of athletes	Gender	Age (yr)	Sport	Positive rate
Grubb (1993)	10	6 M	26 ± 3	Mixed	0/10 (0%)
Manari (1996)	13	11 M	Young	Endurance	3/13 (23%)
Ferrario (1993)	10	10 M	Young	Endurance	5/10 (50%)
Ferrario (1993)	10	10 M	Young	Power	1/10 (10%)
Ferrario (1996)	35	35 M	Young	Mixed	9/35 (26%)

currently possible. Where available (primarily in the United States), mobile cardiac outpatient telemetry may be similarly effective in recording a spontaneous episode. It should be pointed out, however, that none of the available long-term monitoring systems provide insight into the blood pressure.

Permission to compete

Sports eligibility in athletes with a cardiac cause of syncope must be based on the type and severity of the underlying CVD [3–6]. Because of the good prognosis, it appears safe for athletes with NMS to resume competitions, excluding those engaged in potentially traumatic sports during which a disabled athlete might be severely injured [7–10]. Although syncope occurring during effort, compared with those at rest or soon after exercise, tends to be more frequently associated with CVD and almost invariably predicts an unfavorable prognosis, in athletes syncope during physical effort may also be caused by a benign neurally-mediated reflex [7–10]. In these cases, if CVD is excluded by appropriate diagnostic evaluation, athletes may be readmitted to competition. However, treatment of their condition may introduce a problem. Athletes are restricted in the use of certain drugs, several of which are employed for the treatment of NMS; examples include beta-adrenergic blockers (limited in use due to potential for adverse effects on physical performance), alpha agonists, and corticosteroids. Drug restrictions are based on the antidoping rules of the International Olympic Committee. Therefore, a nonpharmacologic therapeutic approach is recommended in these subjects.

Conclusion

The competitive athlete poses an important special circumstance when it comes to evaluating syncope. The physician must not only undertake a very thorough assessment of the individual and devise measures to prevent recurrences, but must also be particularly sensitive in this population to markers suggesting increased risk for sudden death and/or physical injury.

References

1 Kosinski D, Grubb BP, Karas BJ, Frederick S. Exercise-induced neurocardiogenic syncope: clinical data, pathophysiological aspects, and potential role of tilt table test. *Europace* 2000;**2**(1):77–82.
2 Delise P, Guiducci U, Zeppilli P, *et al.* Cardiological guidelines for competitive sports eligibility. *Ital Heart J* 2005;**6**(8):661–702.
3 Mark Estes NA, III, Link MS, Cannom D, *et al.* Report of the NASPE policy conference on arrhythmias and the athlete. *J Cardiovasc Electrophysiol* 2001;**12**:1208–19.
4 Pelliccia A, Fagard R, Bjornstad HH, *et al.* Recommendations for competitive sports participation in athletes with cardiovascular disease. *Eur Heart J* 2005;**26**:1422–45.

5 Zipes DP, Ackerman MJ, Estes NA, III, Grant AO, Myeburg RJ, Van Harre G. 36th Bethesda Conference: Arrhythmias. *J Am Coll Cardiol* 2005;**45**:1354–63.

6 Giada F, Raviele A, Conte R, De Piccoli B. Clinical management of athletes with syncope. *J Sports Cardiol* 2004;**1**:77–83.

7 Calkins H, Seifert M, Morady F. Clinical presentations and long-term follow-up of athletes with exercise-induced vasodepressor syncope. *Am Heart J* 1995;**129**:1159–64.

8 Sakaguchi S, Shultz JJ, Remole SC, Adler SW, Lurie KG, Bendit DG. Syncope associated with exercise, a manifestation of neurally mediated syncope. *Am J Cardiol* 1995;**75**:476–81.

9 Colivicchi F, Ammirati F, Biffi A, Verdile L, Pelliccia A, Santini M. Exercise-related syncope in young competitive athletes without evidence of structural heart disease: clinical presentation and long-term outcome. *Eur Heart J* 2002;**23**(14):1125–30.

10 Colivicchi F, Ammirati F, Santini M. Epidemiology and prognostic implications of syncope in young competing athletes. *Eur Heat J* 2004;**25**:1749–53.

CHAPTER 24

Role of syncope management units

Win K Shen, Michele Brignole

Introduction

The primary difficulty in evaluating patients with syncope in the emergency department (ED) and in the outpatient setting lies in the inherent nature of the condition; i.e., patients are almost always asymptomatic upon arrival. The potential causes of syncope range from benign etiologies to life-threatening arrhythmias [1, 2]. Because a definitive diagnosis often cannot be determined in the time frame available in the ED and the recognition that in some cases syncope may be a harbinger of sudden death among patients with increased risk of cardiogenic causes of syncope, ED physicians generally take a "safe" approach to manage the high- and intermediate-risk patients by admitting most of these patients to the hospital [3–5] when a cause of syncope cannot be immediately established. Although the rationale of this approach is understandable, the presumption that in-hospital evaluation improves a patient's clinical outcome has never been demonstrated. A recent randomized, single-center study [6] showed that a *syncope observational unit* in the ED, with appropriate resources and a multidisciplinary collaboration, could improve the diagnostic yield, reduce hospital admission, and achieve favorable long-term outcome among intermediate-risk patients presented with syncope.

Following hospital admission, concerns of "well-appearing" syncope patients having a "malignant" or adverse outcome frequently result in extensive broad-based evaluations that are often unnecessary and cost-ineffective [7–13]. Two recent prospectively designed observational studies demonstrated improvement of syncope management in the hospital by using a guideline-based decision-making software and a team of syncope-trained personnel in a *syncope management unit* [14, 15]. These are encouraging preliminary evidences supporting efforts in developing and implementing a standardized syncope practice.

In this brief update, drawing references from the last decade, we aim to achieve the following objectives: (1) to provide an overview on risk stratification and the rationale of targeting the intermediate-risk patients in the ED and

Syncope and Transient Loss of Consciousness, 1st edition. Edited by David G Benditt *et al.*
© 2007 Blackwell Publishing, ISBN: 978-1-4051-7625-5.

summarize the European Society of Cardiology (ESC) Syncope Task Force recommendations on when to admit a patient for further evaluation; (2) to review evidence and discuss the current design and utility of a specialized syncope unit in ED and in hospital; (3) to discuss future directions in establishing a guideline-based syncope management unit to improve the effectiveness and efficiency in syncope patient care.

Risk stratification and hospital admission

Risk stratification schemes can be found from the policy statements of the American College of Emergency Physicians (ACEP) [3, 16], from the ESC Syncope Task Force [1, 2], and most recently from a combined statement from the American Heart Association (AHA) and American College of Cardiology Foundation (ACCF), in collaboration with the Heart Rhythm Society (HRS) [17]. In general, clinical and laboratory factors are categorized according to their association with cardiogenic causes of syncope and long-term prognostic outcomes. Patients are usually stratified into three risk categories, as summarized in Table 24.1, depending on their symptoms, signs, laboratory results, and the clinical judgment of the physician [6]. High-risk patients meet the general guidelines [3, 16] for recommendation of hospital admission (ACEP level B recommendation: moderate clinical certainty with class II strength of clinical evidence). Intermediate-risk group meets the general guidelines for "consideration" of hospital admission (level C recommendation: preliminary, inconclusive, or conflicting evidence, or, in the absence of any published data, based on panel consensus). Low-risk patients meet the general guidelines that hospital admission is not required.

The ESC Syncope Task Force has made detailed recommendations on hospital admission (Table 24.2). Nonetheless, many patients who do not have an impending cardiac risk at presentation and do not meet admission guidelines, patients with intermediate or borderline risks are frequently admitted to the hospital [4, 5].

A syncope observational unit in ED

In the Syncope Evaluation in the Emergency Department Study (SEEDS), investigators examined the utility of a critical pathway for the evaluation and management of intermediate-risk patients with syncope presenting to the ED [6]. It was hypothesized that a syncope unit equipped with diagnostic resources that target common causes of syncope would improve the diagnostic yield and reduce the hospital admission rate compared with standard care (controls) at the conclusion of the ED evaluation. The reduction in hospital admission would not negatively affect patient outcomes in survival and recurrent symptoms of syncope.

SEEDS was a prospective, single-center, unblinded randomized study conducted in a tertiary care center in the United States. After initial assessment with a complete history, physical examination, and routine laboratories

Table 24.1 Risk stratification of patients with syncope.*

High-risk group	Intermediate-risk group	Low-risk group
Chest pain compatible with acute coronary syndrome	Age ≥ 50 yr	Age < 50 yr
Signs of congestive heart failure	Previous history of coronary artery disease, myocardial infarction, heart failure, cardiomyopathy without active symptoms, or signs on cardiac medications	With no previous history of cardiovascular disease
Moderate/severe valvular disease		Symptoms consistent with reflex-mediated or vasovagal syncope
History of ventricular arrhythmia	Bundle branch block or Q wave without acute changes on ECG	Normal cardiovascular examination
ECG/cardiac monitor findings of ischemia		Normal ECG findings
Prolonged QTC (<500 ms)	Family history or premature unexplained sudden death (<50 yr)	
Trifascicular block of pauses between 2 and 3 s	Symptoms not consistent with reflex-mediated vasovagal cause	
Third-degree AV block		
Persistent sinus bradycardia between 40 and 60 bpm	Cardiac devices without evidence of dysfunction	
Atrial fibrillation or nonsustained ventricular tachycardia without symptoms	Physician's judgment that a cardiac syncope is possible	
Cardiac devices (pacemaker or defibrillator) with dysfunction		

*This risk stratification scheme was used in the SEEDS.

(electrocardiogram (ECG) and complete blood count), intermediate-risk patients were randomly assigned to standard care or to the syncope unit evaluation. Under the "standard care," patients received continuous cardiac monitoring, nasal oxygen, and intravenous fluid support. Any additional testing in the ED was performed at the discretion of the ED physician on the basis of the patient's initial evaluation. Because of the patient's risk profile and time and resource constraints, most patients in the standard care group were triaged to hospital admission. Patients randomized to the syncope unit evaluation received continuous cardiac telemetry for up to 6 hours, hourly vital signs and orthostatic blood pressure checks, and an echocardiogram for patients with abnormal cardiovascular examination or ECG findings. Tilt-table testing, carotid sinus massage, and electrophysiology consultations were made available to the ED physician. After completion of syncope unit evaluation, a follow-up appointment at one of the outpatient clinics could be arranged, when needed, within 72 hours if the patient is not to be admitted to the

Table 24.2 Hospital admission for syncope management.*

For diagnosis

Strongly recommended
  Suspected or known significant heart disease
  ECG abnormalities suggestive of arrhythmic syncope
  Syncope occurring during exercise
  Syncope causing severe injury
  Strong family history of sudden death

Occasionally may need to be admitted
  Patients with or without heart disease but with:
    • sudden onset of palpitations shortly before syncope
    • syncope in supine position
    • worrisome family history
    • significant physical injury
  Patients with minimal or mild heart disease when there is high suspicion for cardiac syncope

For treatment
  Cardiac arrhythmias as cause of syncope
  Syncope due to cardiac ischemia
  Syncope secondary to the structural cardiac or cardiopulmonary diseases
  Stroke or focal neurologic disorders
  Cardioinhibitory neurally-mediated syncope when a pacemaker implantation is planned

---

*Recommendations from the ESC Syncope Task Force Guidelines.

hospital. These outpatient clinics included, but were not limited to, cardiology, neurology, and general medicine.

The study found that (1) in the ED, a presumptive diagnosis of the cause of syncope was significantly increased from 10% among the "standard care" patients to 67% among those who underwent syncope unit evaluation; (2) hospital admission was reduced from 98% among the standard care patients compared with 43% among the syncope unit patients; (3) the total length of patient-hospital days was reduced by >50% for patients in the syncope unit group; (4) during follow-up, all causes of mortality and recurrent syncope events were similar between the standard care patients and the syncope unit patients. From these results, the investigators concluded that a designated syncope unit in the ED with a multidisciplinary effort and appropriate resources can provide effective and efficient care for a large and challenging group of patients seeking evaluation for syncope. One should be cognizant that the experience from a single-center study may not be generally applied to other hospitals, and the syncope unit has costs of staffing, training, testing, and hospital space. A detailed cost–benefit analysis will be required to assess this novel model for clinical practice in the department.

A syncope management unit in hospital

In the Evaluation of Guidelines in Syncope Study (EGSYS-1), investigators compared the practice patterns among 28 general hospitals in Italy [7]. There was a great degree of both inter- and intradepartmental variability in practice patterns among the hospitals. Although the patient population appeared to be very comparable across all hospitals reviewed, the incidence of admission to the hospital, length of stay, diagnostic tests utilized, and the final presumptive diagnoses were very heterogeneous.

In a follow-up study, these investigators compared six hospitals equipped with a syncope unit organized under the supervision of cardiologists in the hospital to six matched hospitals without such facilities [8]. Although only a small number of patients were referred to the syncope unit in the hospital after ED evaluation, fewer tests and higher number of presumptive diagnoses were observed among patients referred to the syncope unit. In the Osservatorio Epidemiologico della Sincope nel Lazio (OESIL) study, a community hospital-based, prospective, multicenter observational study from the Lazio region of Italy, investigators first reported that some health care delivered to patients with syncope was "inappropriate and ineffective" [9]. In a follow-up study, these investigators implemented a simple two-step diagnostic algorithm from the patient's arrival to ED and throughout the hospital evaluation. The diagnostic algorithm significantly reduced undiagnosed cases from 54 to 18% [10]. From these studies, the same investigators developed a risk score in predicting mortality based on the patient's age, clinical history, presentation, and ECG [11]. In the Epidemiology and Costs of Syncope in Trento (ECSIT) study, a prospective, community-based, single-center study, investigators compared clinical outcomes before and after the implementation of a diagnostic pathway [12]. Although a small reduction in hospital admission was observed (from 53 to 42%), length of hospital stay, number of tests, and costs increased after the implementation of the diagnostic pathway. The investigators concluded that an appropriate and efficacious syncope diagnostic pathway remains far from ideal and simply introducing guidelines may not be sufficient to modify clinical practice. Other studies from the United Kingdom [18] and Austria [19] also made similar observations.

To validate the ESC guidelines on a standardized syncope management pathway, the EGSYS-2 investigators tested the hypothesis that a guideline-based decision-making approach would enhance syncope management in general hospitals [14, 15]. The implementation of this practice was facilitated by using a decision-making software based on the ESC guidelines, a designated physician trained for syncope evaluation, and a central supervisor in each participating hospital. From the 11 Italian general hospitals, these investigators demonstrated that 86% of all study subjects adhered to the guideline-based evaluation, achieving shorter length of hospital stay, fewer diagnostic testing, and higher presumptive diagnoses when compared with the historical controls from the EGSYS-1 study cohort. In a very insightful editorial [13], the author congratulated the EGSYS investigators for this enormous accomplishment in an attempt to establish a standardized syncope evaluation pathway but also provided a few cautions, including the lack of a true control group and a relevant "clinical outcome" end point (ultimately the accurate

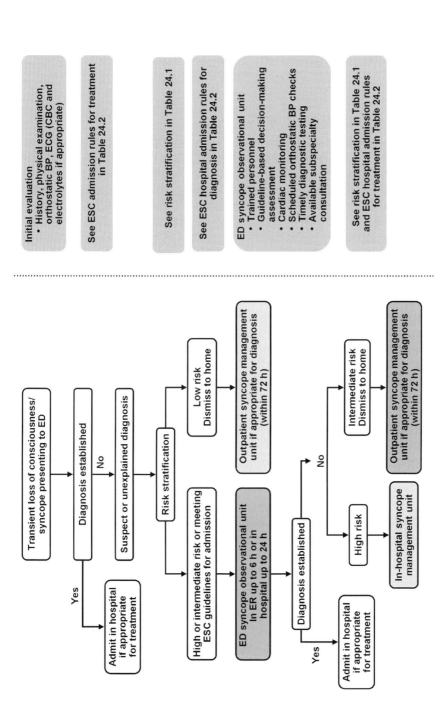

Figure 24.1 The 24-hour hospital syncope unit evaluation proposed here is primarily based on two factors. Within 24 hours, the medical team should aim to draw a decision whether the patient will need to remain in the hospital for further evaluation/therapy or be ready for dismissal and outpatient management. When a hospital stay is less than 24 hours, the patient can be managed under the "observational" status without "being admitted," thereby potentially reducing health care resource utilization.

diagnosis and effective therapy resulting in reduced recurrent syncope), and whether this standardized pathway, requiring significant effort in specialized training of individuals and teams, can be adopted in a universal manner.

Conclusion and future direction

Despite clinical guidelines and consensus statements from ESC, AHA, ACC, HRS, and ACEP, evidence suggests that changes in practice patterns have been slow. Although the cause is certainly complex and multifactorial, heterogeneity of the syncope population and regional differences in clinical practice and available resources are likely major contributors to account for the "lack of progress." Recent data support the notion that a designated syncope management unit, in ED and/or hospital, can provide more efficient and effective triage and evaluation of patients in selected centers. The general strategy in a specialized syncope management unit concept is proposed in Figure 24.1.

Several critical questions remain to be addressed. Is the syncope unit model/critical pathway implemented in SEEDS suitable only in large referral centers with sufficient resources, such as continuous monitoring, availability of cardiac and tilt-table testing, and immediate consultations from electrophysiologists, cardiologists, neurologists, or other subspecialists? Can the training and educational efforts made to the medical staff in the EGSYS-2 be successfully implemented in other hospitals? Should a more "basic" syncope management model suitable for most community hospitals be examined? What additional clinical outcome data may be required to validate a standardized syncope-unit-practice model that can be widely adapted in all hospital practices? Defining and managing the syncope patient with intermediate risk will continue to be a challenge. We anticipate that the syncope management unit concept will continue to evolve and to be refined with additional evidence to eventually provide optimal patient care.

Acknowledgments

We gratefully acknowledge the assistance of Kathy Budensiek and Kate Stai in the preparation of this chapter.

References

1 Brignole M, Alboni P, Benditt DG, *et al.* Guidelines on management (diagnosis and treatment) of syncope. *Eur Heart J* 2001;**22**:1256–306.
2 Brignole M, Alboni P, Benditt DG, *et al.* Guidelines on management (diagnosis and treatment) of syncope—update 2004. *Europace* 2004;**6**:467–537.
3 American College of Emergency Physicians. Clinical policy: critical issues in the evaluation and management of patients presenting with syncope. *Ann Emerg Med* 2001;**37**:771–6.

4 Elesber AA, Decker W, Smars PA, *et al.* Impact of the application of the American College of Emergency Physicians recommendations for the admission of syncopal patients on a retrospectively studied population presenting to the emergency department. *Am Heart J* 2005;**147**:826–31.

5 Bartoletti A, Fabiani P, Adriani P, *et al.* Hospital admission of patients referred to the emergency department for syncope: a single-hospital prospective study based on the application of the European Society of Cardiology guidelines on syncope. *Eur Heart J* 2006;**27**:83–8.

6 Shen WK, Decker WW, Smars P, *et al.* Syncope Evaluation in the Emergency Departments (SEEDS): a multidisciplinary approach to syncope management. *Circulation* 2004;**110**:3636–45.

7 Disertori M, Brignole M, Menozzi C, *et al.* Management of patients with syncope referred urgently to general hospitals. *Europace* 2003;**5**:283–91.

8 Brignole M, Disertori M, Menozzi C, *et al.* Management of syncope referred urgently to general hospitals with and without syncope units. *Europace* 2003;**5**:293–8.

9 Ammirati F, Colivicchi F, Minardi G, *et al.* Hospital management of syncope: the OESIL study (Osservatorio Epidemiologico della Sincope nel Lazio). *G Ital Cardiol* 1999;**29**:533–9.

10 Ammirati F, Colivicchi F, Santini M; on behalf of the Investigators of the OESIL Study. Diagnosing syncope in clinical practice: implementation of a simplified diagnostic algorithm in a multicentre prospective trial—the OESIL 2 study (Osservatorio Epidemiologico della Sincope nel Lazio). *Eur Heart J* 2000;**21**:935–40.

11 Colivicchi F, Ammiati F, Melina D, *et al.* Development and prospective validation of a risk stratification system for patients with syncope in the emergency department: the OESIL risk score. *Eur Heart J* 2003;**24**:822–19.

12 Del Greco M, Cozzio S, Scillieri M, Caprari F, Scivales A, Disertori M; the ECSIT study (Epidemiology and Costs of Syncope in Trento). Diagnostic pathway of syncope and analysis of the impact of guidelines in a district general hospital. *Ital Heart J* 2003;**4**:99–106.

13 Benditt DG. Syncope management guidelines at work: first steps towards assessing clinical utility. *Eur Heart J* 2006;**27**:7–9.

14 Brignole M, Mennozi C, Bartoletti A, *et al.* A new management of syncope: prospective systematic guideline-based evaluation of patients referred urgently to general hospitals. *Eur Heart J* 2006;**27**:76–82.

15 Brignole M, Ungar A, Bartoletti A, *et al.* Standardized-care pathway vs. usual management of syncope patients presenting as emergencies at general hospitals. *Europace* 2006;**8**:644–50.

16 Huff SJ, Decker WW, Quinn JV, *et al.*; for the American College of Emergency Physicians Clinical Policies Subcommittee. Clinical Policy: critical issues in the evaluation and management of adult patients presenting with syncope. *Ann Emerg Med* 2007;**49**:431–44.

17 Strickberger SA, Benson DW, Jr, Biaggioni I, *et al.* AHA/ACCF scientific statement on the evaluation of syncope. *J Am Coll Cardiol* 2006;**47**:473–84.

18 Farwell DJ, Sulke AN. Does the use of a syncope diagnostic protocol improve the investigation and management of syncope? *Heart* 2004;**90**:52–8.

19 Schillinger M, Domanovits H, Mullner M, *et al.* Admission for syncope: evaluation, cost and prognosis. *Wien Klin Wochenschr* 2000;**112**(19):835–41.

CHAPTER 25

The impact of syncope and transient loss of consciousness on quality of life

Blair P Grubb

During the majority of recorded history, physicians have principally concerned themselves with trying to avert death resulting from disease. However, toward the end of the twentieth century there emerged an interest in preserving the "life satisfaction" of patients as well as in the reduction of mortality [1]. This shift in attention came about as a consequence of a tremendous lowering of mortality due to both the wide spread application of public health measures and a dramatic growth in medical science and technology. These changes produced a growing population of individuals with incurable yet chronic diseases, who found themselves "biologically alive and socially dead" [2]. Simultaneously, throughout Western culture there was an increasing concern for personal autonomy and the right of individuals to determine how to live their lives. These concerns led to an interest in systematically measuring (with the hope of improving) the quality of life (QOL) of those suffering from chronic medical illnesses [3]. Defining QOL is challenging, as it is a relatively general concept including "all aspects of life that contribute to its richness, reward, pleasure, and pain" [4]. Thus QOL is deeply influenced by "health," a concept defined by the World Health Organization as "not merely the absence of disease or infirmity" but also a notion that includes a sense of general well-being in all aspects of life (physical, emotional, social, and spiritual).

With these ideas in mind, investigators began to examine the QOL of patients suffering from recurrent episodes of syncope (defined in this chapter somewhat more loosely than in other chapters as the transient loss of consciousness or TLOC). One of the earliest of these studies was that of Linzer and associates [5]. They evaluated the degree of functional impairment in 62 patients with recurrent syncope, using two measures of health status, the sickness impact profile and the symptom checklist 90. They found that function was seriously impaired in patients with recurrent syncope and that the degree of impairment was comparable to that reported in other chronic illnesses, such as rheumatoid arthritis and end-stage renal disease. They also observed that while recurrent

---

Syncope and Transient Loss of Consciousness, 1st edition. Edited by David G Benditt *et al.*
© 2007 Blackwell Publishing, ISBN: 978-1-4051-7625-5.

syncope caused only modest physical impairment, it resulted in a marked degree of psychosocial impairment (similar to that caused by epilepsy).

Later Rose *et al*. evaluated the health-related quality of life (HRQL) in 136 patients with recurrent syncope using the Euro QOL EQ5D as a measure [6]. The EQ5D produces an overall index of health status and classifies HRQL accordingly to five dimensions: mobility, usual activities, self-care, anxiety or depression, and pain or discomfort. They found that HRQL was significantly impaired in syncope patients with more than six lifetime events. They also found that the frequency of syncope affected the HRQL to a greater extent than could be predicted by degree of impairment factor. In contrast to the findings of Linzer, they reported a greater impact of physical impairment on QOL than psychologic impairment in patients with syncope.

Recently, van Dijk *et al*. evaluated 385 patients with recurrent syncope (TLOC), using a Short Form-36 Health Survey and a disease-specific syncope functional status questionnaire [7]. They found that recurrent syncope had a serious effect on QOL, with an average impairment of 33% in all applicable aspects of daily life. Female gender, higher level of comorbidity, duration of complaints, number of syncopal episodes, and the presence of presyncope were all associated with a poorer QOL. Recurrent syncope impaired patient's lives as much as chronic arthritis or moderate depressive disorder.

In reviewing the aforementioned studies, it becomes evident that while the lives of patients suffering from syncope should be relatively normal between events, clearly they are not; the impairment of function and decline in sense of well-being is far beyond that resulting from the syncope itself. These studies also serve to remind us that in clinical medicine we are dealing with people just like ourselves, whose lives have been adversely affected by the medical conditions that affect them, and that our principal role as physicians is to ease human pain and suffering. Thus, the goal in treating patients with recurrent syncope is not solely the prevention of death, but also the maintenance of health and the enrichment of life.

References

1 Armstrong L, Jenkins S. *Every Second Counts*. Broadway Books, New York, 2003: 13.
2 Edmund M, Tancredi LR. Quality of life: an ideological critique. *Perspect Biol Med* 1985;**28**:591–607.
3 Bergner M. Quality of life, health status, and clinical research. *Med Care* 1989;**27**:5148–56.
4 American Thoracic Society. A quality of life resource. Available at www.atsqol.org.
5 Linzer M, Pontinem M, Gold DT, *et al*. Impairment of physical and psychosocial function in recurrent syncope. *J Clin Epidemiol* 1991;**44**:1037–43.
6 Rose MS, Koshman ML, Sprong S, Sheldon R. The relationship between health related quality of life and frequency spells in patients with syncope. *J Clin Epidemiol* 2000;**53**:1209–16.
7 van Dijk N, Sprangers M, Colman N, Boer K, Wieling W, Linzer M. Clinical factors associated with quality of life in patients with transient loss of consciousness. *J Cardiovasc Electrophysiol* 2006;**17**:998–1003.

PART 5

Current controversies and future directions

Driving and flying restrictions for the syncope and/or implanted cardiac device patient

Christina M Murray, Dwight W Reynolds

Introduction

Patients who are at risk for transient loss of consciousness include patients with syncope, nonsyncopal loss of consciousness, and implanted cardiac devices or history of arrhythmias. They constitute a significant number of functional members of society, and many are as active as their disease-free counterparts. For that reason, concerns exist over the safety of those patients and the general public, regarding their participation in activities such as driving and flying. Detailed recommendations have attempted to address these issues [1] as have studies regarding patients in these situations (see Table 26.1).

Driving

In the United States, state laws, in accordance with individual physician recommendations, govern licensing for driving. For syncope patients, recommendations from the European Society of Cardiology (ESC) are classified according to the type of syncope and control of symptoms, based on 2004 updated recommendations [2], and are similar to those proposed by the Heart Rhythm Society [1].

Syncope is a term with broad implications, and with respect to driving, most forms are similarly managed. For single episode or mild vasovagal or carotid sinus syncope, no restrictions are imposed, and for those with severe symptoms, driving is restricted until symptoms are controlled. Situational syncope of mild nature has no restrictions, whereas severe symptoms mandate disqualification until appropriate therapy is established.

Even for commercial drivers with mild/single-episode syncope, no restriction is imposed, unless symptoms occurred in high-risk driving situations. In those with severe syncope, permanent restriction is recommended unless

Syncope and Transient Loss of Consciousness, 1st edition. Edited by David G Benditt *et al.*
© 2007 Blackwell Publishing, ISBN: 978-1-4051-7625-5.

Table 26.1 Suggested restrictions for syncope and device patients.

	Driving	Flying
Syncope patients	• Single or mild episode—no restriction • Severe or recurrent symptoms—restricted driving until symptoms controlled • Applies to commercial and private drivers	• Disqualifying medical condition • May apply for special issuance, with medical record review by panel • Should have 1–2-yr syncope-free period
Pacemaker patients	• No restriction if arrhythmia is controlled • Applies to commercial and private drivers	• Disqualifying medical condition • May apply for special issuance, with medical record review by panel
ICD patients	• Primary prevention patients—restricted in acute healing phase only • Secondary prevention—6 mo from implant (no events) or 6 mo event free • Primary experiencing shock—treat as secondary • Cannot be certified for commercial driving	• Permanently disqualified

effective treatment has been established. For those with syncope of uncertain cause, restriction is appropriate until diagnosis is established and therapy is under way.

Pacemaker patients have no restriction as long as the patient is not pacemaker dependent. In cases where they are pacemaker dependent, they should have a period of restriction, until follow-up assures adequate protection from adverse symptoms [1].

Implantable cardioverter-defibrillator (ICD) patients represent another group that is potentially at risk while driving, both from syncope and other symptoms associated with malignant ventricular arrhythmias and from shock therapy. In the lowest risk patient group to date, Sudden Cardiac Death in Heart Failure Trial (SCD-HeFT), a study involving patients having ICDs implanted as primary prevention therapy for sudden cardiac arrest (SCA), the annual rate of shocks was 7.5% [3]. Selected secondary prevention groups will have higher rates. Triggers of Ventricular Arrhythmias (TOVA) study, an ICD cohort study (patients with a 1998 class I or IIa ICD indication, $n = 1140$), reported higher rates of ICD shocks based on clinical status, including lower ejection fraction and clinical heart failure, with an annual risk of 12.1% for those with clinical heart failure and 6.5% for those without [4]. Arguably, patients may be at a higher risk for shocks in the first months after implant [5]. In Arrhythmics Versus Implantable Defibrillators (AVID) trial patients, a secondary SCA prevention trial, resumption of driving was common (57% by 3 months and 78% by 6 months), with restriction by physician being the most common reason for not driving [6]. There were notable events in that population while driving: 8% had a shock while driving, 2% suffered loss of consciousness while driving, 11% had dizziness or palpitations that necessitated stopping the vehicle, and 22% had dizziness or palpitations that did not require stopping the vehicle. Auto accidents were experienced at a rate of 3.4% per patient-year, compared with 6.2% in the same patients in the preceding year, which is consistent with the US Federal Statistic of 7.1% in the general population reported in the same article.

HRS [7] and ESC put forth very similar recommendations for ICD patients regarding driving. Primary SCA prevention patients should not be restricted from driving except during the acute healing phase, 1 week after implant. In this period, potential system complications may become apparent. If patients remain asymptomatic from an arrhythmia standpoint, no further restrictions are suggested. If a shock is received from a primary prevention device, the patient should be transitioned from primary to secondary prevention guidelines, and a period of restricted driving for 6 months may be appropriate. The HRS guidelines indicate the importance of consideration of other medical conditions that may compromise driving ability (angina and heart failure symptoms), and the importance of notifying the patient that impairment of consciousness may be possible.

Flying

The acquisition of a new or renewed pilot's license by a syncope or device patient may be considerably more challenging than is obtaining driving permission. In the United States, Federal Aviation Administration (FAA) (http://www.faa.gov/about/office_org/headquarters_offices/avs/offices/aam/ame/guide/app_process/general/decision/) typically regards conditions such as disturbance of consciousness, permanent cardiac pacemaker (or ICD), coronary artery disease with angina or past treatment, and valve replacement as disqualifying medical conditions. Pilots' licenses, whether commercial or private, are bound by the same restrictions. These are perhaps more stringently applied in the case of commercial pilots. Special issuances of licenses may be obtained with an application process requiring extensive medical record review.

Following are some situations that are typically encountered by the FAA medical decision panels (Eliot Schechter, personal communication). In the case of cardiology review, cases are reviewed by four to six cardiologists who serve on a medical decision panel. An additional panel (e.g., neurologic) may be relevant in individual cases. If there is a reasonable explanation indicating that syncope is unlikely to occur during flying (e.g., vasovagal syncope with phlebotomy), the pilot may return to flying status. Unexplained syncope carries a requirement for a 1–2-year syncope-free observation period before returning to flying. Pacemaker and ICD patients are also given careful scrutiny. The presence of an ICD is considered a disqualifying condition. The logic of this is twofold. Both the risk of loss of consciousness and the inability to control an aircraft while receiving ICD therapy or shocks are felt to preclude safe operation of the aircraft. While a pacemaker is considered a disqualifying condition, a special issuance is possible. Pacemaker patients are required to have a 2-month recovery period and then they may be eligible if not in precarious health or pacemaker dependent.

Conclusion

Driving motor vehicles and flying aircraft represent special challenges for patients with a history of susceptibility to syncope and/or other forms of transient loss of consciousness, as well as for patients in whom pacemakers and defibrillators have been implanted. Issues involve protecting not only the patients but also the public at potential risk.

Government agency regulations vary among geographies and will need to be consulted by physicians responsible for individual patient care. Generally, patients with mild or isolated symptoms are reasonably unrestricted with respect to driving and flying, whereas patients with more severe, recurrent, and/or unexplained symptoms are restricted. Patients with pacemakers and ICDs are special cases with, appropriately or inappropriately, more restrictions placed for the latter, especially for flying aircraft.

References

1 Epstein AE, Miles WM, Benditt DG, et al. Personal and public safety issues related to arrhythmias that may affect consciousness: implications for regulation and physician recommendations: a medical/scientific statement from the American Heart Association and the North American Society of pacing and electrophysiology. Circulation 1996;94:1147–66.

2 Brignole M, Alboni P, Benditt DG, et al.; Task Force on Syncope, European Society of Cardiology. Guidelines on management (diagnosis and treatment) of syncope: Executive Summary. Eur Heart J 2004;25:2054–72.

3 Bardy GH, Lee KL, Mark DB, et al. Amiodarone or an implantable cardioverter-defibrillator for congestive heart failure. N Engl J Med 2005;352:225–37.

4 Whang W, Mittleman MA, Rich DQ, et al. Heart failure and the risk of shocks in patients with implantable cardioverter defibrillators: results from the triggers of ventricular arrhythmias (TOVA) study. Circulation 2004;1009:1386–91.

5 Larsen GC, Stupey MR, Walance CG, et al. Recurrent cardiac events in survivors of ventricular fibrillation or tachycardia: implications for driving restrictions. JAMA 1994;271:1335–9.

6 Akiyama T, Powell JL, Mitchell LB, et al. Resumption of driving after life-threatening ventricular tachyarrhythmia. N Engl J Med 2001;345:391–7.

7 Epstein AE, Baessler CA, Curtis AB, et al. Addendum to "personal and public safety issues related to arrhythmias that may affect consciousness: implications for regulation and physician recommendations: a medical/scientific statement from the AHA/NASPE." Heart Rhythm 2007;4:1–6.

CHAPTER 27

Clinical trials landscape: what's new, what's ongoing, what do we need

Michele Brignole, David G Benditt, Wouter Wieling

Introduction

Randomized clinical trials usually offer little by way of scientific novelty. Nevertheless, they have become an essential element of the assessment of new diagnostic and therapeutic techniques. In particular, the double-blind, randomized clinical trial (RCT) ranks highest in the hierarchy of medical evidence. Where possible, relying on RCT-confirmed observations is the most reliable approach to the care of patients, including those with apparent transient loss of consciousness (TLOC)/syncope. However, as is true throughout medicine, RCTs addressing a particular clinical issue are often not available. In such circumstances, less rigorous studies, or even expert consensus, continue to be valuable aids to the clinician.

This chapter summarizes the most important controlled trials published related to the management of syncope since the 2004 ESC Syncope Guideline update. Our goal is to provide the readers the most recent clinical evidence upon which to base their clinical practice and to illustrate the direction of current thinking.

What's new?

Since publication of the ESC Syncope Guidelines in 2004, around 1700 new articles related to syncope have been cited in Medline (period January 2004–March 2007). Some of these reports describe controlled clinical trials that are likely to change the practice and therefore find a place in upcoming guidelines. These latter reports form the focus of this update.

Further evidence of failure of pharmacologic therapy (metoprolol, salt, and fludrocortisone) to prevent syncopal recurrences in patients with vasovagal syncope

Metoprolol was not effective in preventing vasovagal syncope in the placebo-controlled, double-blind Prevention of Syncope Trial (POST) [1]. Patients

Syncope and Transient Loss of Consciousness, 1st edition. Edited by David G Benditt *et al.*
© 2007 Blackwell Publishing, ISBN: 978-1-4051-7625-5.

received either metoprolol at highest tolerated doses from 25 to 200 mg daily or a matching placebo. The main outcome measure was the first recurrence of syncope. A total of 208 patients (mean age 42 ± 18 yr) with a median of nine syncopal spells over a median of 11 years were randomized. Randomization was stratified according to ages <42 and >42 years.

There were 75 patients with more than one syncope recurrence over a 1-year treatment period. The likelihood of recurrent syncope was not significantly different between groups. Also, the age of the patient did not predict subsequent significant benefit from metoprolol.

Salt and fludrocortisone were not effective in preventing vasovagal syncope in one recent placebo-controlled, double-blind trial in children [2]. Thirty-three tilt-positive children (mean age 13.9 ± 2.5 yr) with syncope or severe presyncope were randomized to receive either fludrocortisone 0.1 mg/day and salt 1 g/day or placebo two capsules per day for 1 year. The number of syncopal episodes before therapy was 4.4 ± 4.8. Therapy was continued for 176 ± 117 days. Symptoms recurred in 10 of 18 children on fludrocortisone and salt and in 5 of 14 children on placebo ($p < 0.04$). Children on placebo had no symptoms until they discontinued their study medications. These data raise the potential of a significant placebo effect with pharmacologic therapy. A trial with fludrocortisone in adults is currently ongoing (see below).

Physical counterpressure therapies are effective in preventing syncopal recurrences in patients with vasovagal syncope. Uncertainty still persists for tilt training

Leg and arm counterpressure maneuvers (leg crossing, handgripping, and arm tensing) should be advised as first-line treatment in patients presenting with vasovagal syncope with prodromal symptoms. The multicenter, prospective, randomized Physical Counterpressure (PC) trial [3] assessed the effectiveness of physical counterpressure maneuvers (PCM) in daily life in 223 patients, aged 38 ± 15 years, with recurrent vasovagal syncope and a recognizable prodromal (i.e., warning) symptoms: 117 patients were randomized to standardized conventional therapy alone, and 106 patients received conventional therapy plus training in counterpressure maneuvers. The median yearly syncope burden during follow-up was significantly lower in the group trained in PCM than in the control group ($p < 0.004$); overall 51% of the patients with conventional treatment and 32% of the patients trained in PCM experienced a syncopal recurrence ($p < 0.005$). Actuarial recurrence-free survival was better in the treatment group (log-rank $p < 0.018$), resulting in a relative risk reduction of 39% (95% CI 11–53). No adverse events were reported.

A recent study [4] suggests that lower limb compression bandaging is effective in diminishing orthostatic systolic blood fall and reducing symptoms in elderly patients affected by progressive orthostatic hypotension. Progressive orthostatic hypotension is a common problem in the elderly because of age-related impairment in baroreflex-mediated vasoconstriction and chronotropic responses of the heart, as well as the deterioration of the diastolic filling of the heart. The rationale for the use of elastic compression bandages is to apply an external counterpressure to the capacitance beds of abdomen and legs in order to improve the venous return to the heart. In the acute tilt-table study, 21 patients (mean age 70 ± 11 yr) underwent two tilt-table test procedures, with and without elastic bandage of the legs (compression pressure 40–60 mmHg) and of the abdomen (compression pressure 20–30 mmHg) in a randomized crossover fashion. Leg bandage was administered for 10 minutes and followed by additional abdominal bandage for an additional 10 minutes. In the placebo arm, systolic blood pressure decreased from 125 ± 18 mmHg immediately after tilting to 112 ± 25 mmHg after 10 minutes of placebo leg bandaging and to 106 ± 25 mmHg after 20 minutes, despite the addition of placebo abdominal bandaging. The corresponding values with active therapy were 129 ± 19, 127 ± 17 ($p = 0.003$ vs placebo), and 127 ± 21 ($p = 0.002$ vs placebo) respectively. In the active arm, 90% of patients remained asymptomatic, versus 53% in the control arm ($p = 0.02$). Irrespective of the results of the acute tilt phase, all patients were trained to wear daily elastic leg-compression stockings. The elastic leg-compression stockings were chosen, among those commonly available in stores, to have a nominal degree of compression of 40–60 mmHg at the level of the ankles and 30–40 mmHg at the hip level. In this uncontrolled clinical follow-up feasibility study, home treatment based on self-administered elastic leg-compression stockings was feasible, safe, and well accepted by the majority of the patients. After a 6-month follow-up, two-thirds of the patients continued to wear the elastic stockings, declared them to be comfortable, and were satisfied with that therapy. As a consequence, the symptom burden of the patients decreased approximately 37% (from 35 points baseline of the specific symptom scale to 22.5 points after 1 month of therapy, $p = 0.01$). However, longer follow-up periods are needed to assess tolerance and effectiveness.

Two randomized controlled trials [5, 6] failed to confirm short-term effectiveness of tilt training in reducing the positive response rate of tilt-table test. In the multicenter Italian trial [5], 62 patients with recurrent neurally-mediated reflex syncope and two positive nitroglycerin-potentiated head-up tilt tests were randomized to tilt training or no treatment. The tilt-training program consisted of daily 30-minute sessions of upright standing against a vertical wall, 6 days a week for at least 3 weeks, until a reevaluation tilt test. On this third head-up tilt test, 19 (59%) of 32 tilt-trained patients and 18 (60%) of 30 controls still had a positive test. Treated patients performed a mean number of 15 ± 7 sessions but only 11 patients (34%) did all the programmed sessions. In the single-center Korean trial [6], 42 tilt-positive patients were randomized to home tilt training for 7 days a week for 4 weeks or an untreated control arm. After this period, 9 of 16 tilt-trained patients (56%) had a positive tilt response versus 9 of 17 untreated controls (53%).

A key limitation of these studies is the use of tilt-table testing as an end point. A large randomized study using a hard clinical end point (i.e., syncope) seems advisable before making any conclusion on efficacy of such physical therapy.

Specific therapy guided by implantable loop recorder is effective in preventing syncopal recurrences in patients with suspected neurally-mediated syncope

A strategy based on early application of an implantable loop recorder (ILR) with therapy delayed until documentation of syncope allows a safe, specific, and effective therapy for patients with recurrent suspected neurally-mediated syncope. The International Study on Syncope of Uncertain Etiology 2 (ISSUE-2) study [7] was a multicenter, prospective, controlled study enrolling patients with a diagnosis of suspected neurally-mediated syncope (made in accordance with the guidelines of the European Society of Cardiology), early ILR placement, and ILR-based specific therapy after syncope recurrence. In ISSUE-2, 53 patients received ILR-based specific therapy, mostly pacemaker therapy ($n = 47$), and 50 patients received counseling (education and reassurance). Patient characteristics were well matched for the two groups. The 1-year recurrence rate in patients assigned to a specific therapy was 10% (burden 0.07 ± 0.2 episodes per patient per year) compared with 41% (burden 0.83 ± 1.57 episodes per patient per year) in the patients without specific therapy (80% relative risk reduction for patients, $p = 0.002$, and 92% for burden, $p = 0.002$). The 1-year recurrence rate in patients with pacemakers was 5% (burden 0.05 ± 0.15 episodes per patient per year). Severe trauma secondary to syncope relapse occurred in 2% and mild trauma in 4% of the patients during the overall study period.

New prolonged ECG monitoring systems can be regarded as the reference standard for the diagnosis of arrhythmic syncope

Knowledge of what occurs during a spontaneous syncopal episode is currently the gold standard for arrhythmic syncope evaluation. The diagnostic value of provocative laboratory testing can be evaluated against this gold standard.

Head-up tilt-table testing and the adenosine triphosphate test (ATP) have not proved as effective for predicting the mechanism of spontaneous symptoms in patients with neurally-mediated syncope as initially hoped. Therefore, while these tests may have diagnostic utility, they are of uncertain value in guiding specific therapy.

In the ISSUE-2 diagnosis study [8], 343 patients underwent tilt-table testing which was positive in 164 (48%) individuals. In addition, 180 patients underwent an ATP, which was positive in 53 (29%) cases. Syncope was documented by an ILR in 106 (26%) patients at a median of 3-month follow-up. Patients with positive and negative tilt-table tests had similar baseline characteristics, syncopal recurrence rate, and apparent mechanism of syncope. An asystolic pause was more frequently found during spontaneous syncope than during tilt-table testing (45% vs 21%, $p = 0.02$), but there was a trend for those with an asystolic response on tilt-table test also to have an asystolic response during spontaneous syncope (75% vs 37%, $p = 0.1$). Patients with positive ATP responses showed syncopal recurrence rates and apparent mechanism of syncope similar to those with negative ATPs. These results are consistent with those of two previous smaller studies [9, 10].

In the Eastbourne Syncope Assessment Study (EaSyAS) trial [11], 201 patients (median age 74 yr) with recurrent unexplained syncope were randomized to receive an ILR or conventional investigation and management. During a median follow-up of 17 months, 42 (43%) ILR patients and 8 (6%) conventional group patients received an ECG diagnosis (hazard ratio 6.53, 95% CI 3.73–11.4, $p < 0.001$). ECG-directed therapy was commenced in 43 and 7 patients respectively in the two groups resulting in a longer time to second syncope for the ILR group ($p < 0.04$).

Telemedicine will become increasingly important for the identification of clinically significant but infrequent, brief, and/or intermittently symptomatic arrhythmias. The new mobile cardiac outpatient telemetry system (MCOT, Cardionet Inc, San Diego, CA) provided a significantly higher yield when compared with a patient-activated external looping event monitor (LOOP) in a 17-center prospective clinical trial with patients randomized to either LOOP or MCOT for up to 30 days [12]. A total of 266 patients who completed the monitoring period were analyzed. A diagnosis was made in 88% of MCOT subjects compared with 75% of LOOP subjects ($p = 0.008$). In a subgroup of patients presenting with syncope or presyncope, a diagnosis was made in 89% of MCOT subjects versus 69% of LOOP subjects ($p = 0.008$). MCOT was superior in confirming the diagnosis of clinically significant arrhythmias, detecting such events in 55 of 134 patients (41%) compared with 19 of 132 patients (15%) in the LOOP group ($p < 0.001$). The MCOT system was also evaluated in a separate observational study that showed similar results [13]. Currently, MCOT is available only in the United States but should become more widely available in the future.

Standardized guideline-based care pathways improve diagnostic yield and reduce hospital admissions and resource consumption compared with conventional evaluation

Some controlled trials showed that a standardized guideline-based care pathway significantly improved diagnostic yield and reduced hospital admissions, resource consumption, and overall costs. Thus, they support the creation of cohesive, structured syncope facilities, which are organized to provide optimal quality service on the basis of well-defined up-to-date diagnostic guidelines. Two different models of syncope facilities have been developed, one primarily centered within emergency departments ("asyncope observation unit") and the other within the cardiology department ("syncope management unit").

The *syncope observation unit* operating primarily in conjunction with an emergency department has as its principal goal to risk-stratify patients and to define the appropriate care pathways. The Syncope Evaluation in the Emergency Department Study (SEEDS) [14] evaluated the hypothesis that a designated syncope unit in the emergency department improves diagnostic yield and reduces hospital admission for patients with syncope who are at intermediate risk for an adverse cardiovascular outcome according to the Guidelines on Syncope of the American College of Emergency Physicians. In this prospective single-center study, patients were randomly allocated to two treatment arms: syncope unit evaluation and standard care. The study enrolled 103 individuals. Fifty-one patients were randomized to the syncope observation unit care. In terms of outcomes, comparing syncope observation unit versus standard care patients, a presumptive diagnosis was established in 34 (67%) and 5 (10%) patients respectively, and hospital admission was required for 22 (43%) and 51 (98%) patients, respectively. With the observation unit, total patient-hospital days were reduced from 140 to 64. Thus, the novel syncope observation unit designed for this study significantly improved diagnostic yield in the emergency department and reduced hospital admission and total length of hospital stay.

In another emergency department based study, the "San Francisco Syncope Rule" was applied [15]. This rule employs an abnormal ECG, a complaint of shortness of breath, hematocrit <30%, systolic blood pressure <90 mmHg, or a history of congestive heart failure as markers in order to risk-stratify patients and improve the use of hospital admission. The rule was 98% sensitive and 56% specific to predict serious outcomes (defined as death, myocardial infarction, arrhythmia, pulmonary embolism, stroke, subarachnoid hemorrhage, significant hemorrhage, or any condition causing a return emergency department visit and hospitalization in 791 patients referred to the emergency department of a teaching hospital). However, in one external validation cohort [16] the San Francisco Syncope Rule had a lower sensitivity and specificity than in previous reports (89 and 42%).

The *syncope management unit* model adopted in some Italian hospitals is a functional unit managed by cardiologists inside the department of cardiology, with dedicated medical and support personnel. The patients attending this syncope unit have preferential access to all the other facilities and investigations within the department, including admission to cardiology wards or the intensive care unit if indicated. Where appropriate, patients are jointly managed with other specialists. The patients are referred to the unit from the emergency department, as well from inpatient or outpatient clinics. However, the personnel of the unit are not usually involved in the "initial evaluation" of the patient.

In the context of more structured approach to the syncope evaluation, EGSYS-2 [17] examined a decision-making approach based on adherence to the recommendations of the updated guidelines of the European Society of Cardiology. A prospective, controlled, multicenter study was performed in order to verify if this standardized method of care is superior to the usual care [18]. There were 929 patients in the usual care and 745 patients in the standardized care group. The baseline characteristics of the two study populations were similar. At the end of the evaluation, compared to usual care, the standardized care group resulted in 17% lower hospitalization rate (39% vs 47%), 11% shorter in-hospital stay (7.2 ± 5.7 days vs 8.1 ± 5.9 days), and 26% fewer tests performed per patient (median 2.5 vs 3.4). Forty-one percent more standardized care patients had a diagnosis of neurally-mediated syncope (65% vs 46%), 66% more of orthostatic syncope (10% vs 6%), 54% fewer had a diagnosis of pseudosyncope (6% vs 13%), and 75% fewer of unexplained syncope (5% vs 20%). The mean cost per patient was 19% lower (€1127 vs €1394), and the mean cost per diagnosis was 29% lower (€1240 vs €1753) in the standardized care group.

What's ongoing?

A number of ongoing trials are addressing important points regarding the efficacy of certain proposed therapies for neurally-mediated syncope (fludrocortisone, midodrine, hydratation, and cardiac pacing), as well as the validation of standardized management pathways. Some of these are given in Table 27.1.

What do we need?

To define the diagnostic value (sensitivity, specificity, and predictive value) and cost-effectiveness of the conventional investigations and develop a standardized validated diagnostic pathway

Ultimately, technology may allow recording of multiple signals in addition to the ECG (e.g., blood flow or pressure and EEG) and the automatic immediate wireless transmission of pertinent data to a central monitoring station. Such advances will permit greater emphasis on the documentation and characterization of spontaneous symptom episodes. The diagnostic value of conventional investigations (initial evaluation and provocative laboratory testing) could then be validated against this "ideal" gold standard of prolonged multisystem monitoring.

To assess the prognostic value determined by occurrence of syncope in patients with inherited syndromes (e.g., long QT syndrome and Brugada syndrome) and to assess the benefit of specific therapy, i.e., implantable cardioverter-defibrillator, by means of controlled trials

In existing trials the prognostic value of syncope has been investigated as part of multiple risk factor evaluation. A confounding effect was that syncope was frequently used as a covariate risk factor when syncope was also used as an end-point event. As consequence, the efficacy of therapy, i.e., implantable cardioverter-defibrillator (ICD), in patients with syncope is not yet proven. Some examples are as follows:

• In a large multicenter prospective observational trial [19] performed on 812 adult patients affected by long QT syndrome (LQTS), the cardiac event end points included syncope (transient abrupt onset and offset of loss of consciousness), cardiac arrest (requiring defibrillation), and LQTS-related sudden death. These end points occurred in 192 (23%) patients. When syncope was removed from end points, cardiac arrest and sudden death occurred in only 50 (6%) patients, showing that syncope is three times more frequent than the other

Table 27.1 Ongoing trials on syncope.

Acronym/principal investigator/clinical Trials. gov identifier	Title	Study description	Follow-up duration	Primary endpoint	Number of patients	Study start/ expected study end
POST 2 Sheldon* NCT00118482	A randomized clinical trial of fludrocortisone for vasovagal syncope: the Second Prevention of Syncope Trial (POST II)	Treatment, randomized, double-blind, placebo-controlled, parallel assignment	12 mo	Time to first recurrence of syncope	310	2005/2010
Kaufmann H NCT00004479	Randomized study of midodrine, an alpha-adrenergic agonist, in patients with neurally-mediated syncope	Treatment, randomized, double-blind, crossover, placebo-controlled study	—	—	—	Completed, not yet published
STAND Wieling	Midodrine in patients who fail conventional therapy including physical maneuvers	Treatment, randomized, double-blind	—	Syncope recurrence	—	—
Leftheriotis NCT00143754	Benefit of controlled rehydration in unexplained syncope	Randomized, single-blind, uncontrolled, parallel assignment	—	—	—	2005/Completed not yet published
ISSUE 3 Brignole† NCT00359203	Pacemaker therapy for patients with asystolic neurally-mediated syncope	Treatment, randomized, double-blind, placebo-controlled, parallel assignment (after asystolic syncope documentation by ILR)	24 mo	Time to first recurrence of syncope	710	2006/2009
SCANSYNC Mølgaard NCT00292825	Effect of closed loop pacemaker treatment on recurrent vasovagal syncope	Treatment, randomized, double-blind, placebo-controlled, crossover assignment	12 + 12 mo	Time to first recurrence of syncope	100	2006/2009
ELIAS Ehlers NCT00170261	Early loop-recorder in suspected arrhythmogenic syncope	Diagnostic, randomized, open label, active control, parallel assignment (early loop-recorder vs conventional investigations)	—	Cost of diagnostics per patient until final cardiac diagnosis has been made	100	2002/-
SUP Brignole	A prospective systematic guideline-based evaluation and treatment of patients referred to the syncope units of general hospitals	Observational longitudinal, prospective study in patients with syncope referred to a syncope unit	12 mo	ESC guidelines validation	600	2007/2009
Adrienne J Birnbaum NCT00300625	Validation of the San Francisco Syncope Rule	Observational longitudinal, prospective study in patients with acute syncope or near syncope as a reason for the ED visit	1 mo	Identify patients with a serious outcome	—	2005/-
NINDS NCT00069693	Evaluation of chronic orthostatic intolerance	Observational	—	Natural history	200	2003/-

* Brignole *et al. Europace* 2007;**9**:25–30.
† Raj *et al. Am Heart J* 2006;**151**:1186.e11–7.

end points. Therefore, in this setting, it seems that syncope does not necessarily carry a high risk of major life-threatening cardiac events. On the other hand, syncope was associated with a significant fivefold increased risk of cardiac arrest or sudden death, which occurred in a minority of patients. In other words, as a marker for life-threatening events, syncope has low sensitivity. The likely conclusion is that the mechanism of syncope in LQTS patients may be heterogeneous, being caused by life-threatening arrhythmias in some, but being of a more benign origin, i.e., vasovagal, in many others. Consequently, even in LQTS there is a need for more precise diagnosis of the mechanism of syncope.

• The same reasoning applies to the patients with the ECG Brugada pattern who have a history of syncope. In a multicenter study [20], 40% of 220 Brugada patients implanted with an ICD had a history of syncope, but the patients with syncope were not at a higher risk of appropriate ICD discharge than those who had been asymptomatic. Similarly, in a single-center study [21], a history of syncope was present in 55% of 47 patients who received an ICD but was unrelated to appropriate ICD discharge; one might reasonably infer from these observations that the likely diagnosis in those who had syncope relapse after the ICD implantation was vasovagal and not a potentially life-threatening arrhythmia. Finally, in a large meta-analysis [22] encompassing 1140 patients (262 of them (23%) with a history of syncope), the patients with syncope had the same risk of ventricular tachyarrhythmias as those who had been without syncope and significantly lower than those presenting with documented cardiac arrest.

To assess the prognostic value determined by occurrence of syncope in patients with structural heart disease and assess the benefit of specific therapy, i.e., ICD, by means of controlled trials

Frequent errors in syncope management include confounding the prognostic significance of syncope with that of the underlying heart disease and mistaking the therapy of syncope with the therapy of the underlying heart disease. An ICD is recommended in patients with syncope and structural heart disease with ejection fraction <30% independently of the cause of syncope. An ICD would be indicated even in the absence of syncope for the underlying structural heart disease, and so the role of syncope in the decision-making process is uncertain. Conversely, the additive prognostic value of syncope in patients with less severe systolic dysfunction is uncertain, as well as the efficacy of an empiric ICD implantation compared with a mechanism-guided specific therapy.

To evaluate the efficacy of any therapy of neurally-mediated syncope by means of double-blind, randomized controlled trials

In general, while the results have been satisfactory in uncontrolled trials or short-term controlled trials, several long-term placebo-controlled prospective trials have been unable to show a benefit of the active drug over placebo with few exceptions. For instance, no large RCT has been performed in patients affected by carotid sinus syndrome in order to evaluate the effect of cardiac pacing; the efficacy of tilt training is not yet proven by a large RCT; elastic stocking of the leg and abdomen has been shown to be effective in acute or noncontrolled follow-up studies but still requires confirmation of efficacy by RCT, etc.

Conclusion

Before an idea can be confirmed or quantified by controlled trials, it must have a convincing scientific background based on pathophysiology, epidemiology, and diagnostic testing. In this regard there remain many areas of interest that still require investigations, such as:
• Understanding the difference between the pathophysiology of isolated vaso-vagal syncope (which typically occurs in the young) from a condition that might be termed vasovagal "disease" (which typically occurs in the elderly). Inasmuch as vasovagal susceptibility is probably present in all healthy humans, isolated vasovagal syncope is a physiological phenomenon. This event occurs in patients whose autonomic regulation outside the episodes of syncope is normal. Vasovagal disease, on the other hand, begins in the advanced age of diseased patients. In vasovagal disease, outside the episodes of syncope autonomic regulation is usually not normal [23].
• Obtaining comprehensive epidemiological data on syncope (including its impact on quality of life and the interrelationship with psychological factors) from unselected general population. Some data suggest a bimodal presentation of syncope with a first peak around 15–25 years and a second peak over 70 years [23]. Some familiar predisposition to fainting has recently been shown [24].

In closing, it is evident that careful study has contributed importantly to improving our understanding of the TLOC/syncope syndrome, and best approaches to its management. However, it must be equally clear that not every element of syncope/TLOC care can be subjected to RCT testing. The important role of expert consensus opinion both in day-to-day care and in practice guideline development will remain a critical part of the landscape for a long time to come.

References

1 Sheldon R, Connolly S, Rose S, *et al.*; POST Investigators. Prevention of Syncope Trial (POST): a randomized, placebo-controlled study of metoprolol in the prevention of vaso-vagal syncope. *Circulation* 2006;**113**:1164–70.
2 Salim MA, Di Sessa TG. Effectiveness of fludrocortisone and salt in preventing syncope recurrence in children: a double-blind, placebo-controlled, randomized trial. *J Am Coll Cardiol* 2005;**45**:484–8.

3 van Dijk N, Quartieri F, Blanc JJ, *et al*. Effectiveness of physical counterpressure maneuvers in preventing vasovagal syncope: the physical counterpressure maneuvres trial (PC-trial). *J Am Coll Cardiol* 2006;**48**:1652–7.

4 Podoleanu C, Maggi R, Brignole M, *et al*. Lower limb and abdominal compression bandages prevent progressive orthostatic hypotension in the elderly: a randomized placebo-controlled study. *J Am Coll Cardiol* 2006;**48**:1425–32.

5 Foglia-Manzillo G, Giada F, Gaggioli G, *et al*. Efficacy of tilt training in the treatment of neurally mediated syncope: a randomized study. *Europace* 2004;**6**:199–204.

6 Keun On Y, Park J, Huh J, *et al*. Is home orthostatic self-training effective in preventing neurocardiogenic syncope? A prospective and randomized study. *Pacing Clin Electrophysiol* 2007. In press.

7 Brignole M, Sutton R, Menozzi C, *et al*. Early application of an implantable loop recorder allows a mechanism-based effective therapy in patients with recurrent suspected neurally-mediated syncope. *Eur Heart J* 2006;**27**:1085–92.

8 Brignole M, Sutton R, Menozzi C, *et al*. Lack of correlation between the responses to tilt testing and adenosine triphosphate test and the mechanism of spontaneous neurally-mediated syncope. *Eur Heart J* 2006;**27**:2232–9.

9 Donateo P, Brignole M, Menozzi C, *et al*. Mechanism of syncope in patients with positive adenosine triphosphate tests. *J Am Coll Cardiol* 2003;**41**:93–8.

10 Deharo JC, Jego C, Lanteaume A, *et al*. An implantable loop recorder study of highly symptomatic vasovagal patients: the heart rhythm observed during a spontaneous syncope is identical to the recurrent syncope but not correlated with the head-up tilt test or ATP test. *J Am Coll Cardiol* 2006;**47**:587–93.

11 Farwell DJ, Freemantle N, Sulke N. The clinical impact of implantable loop recorders in patients with syncope. *Eur Heart J* 2006;**27**:351–6.

12 Rothman SA, Laughlin JC, Seltzer J, *et al*. The diagnosis of cardiac arrhythmias: a prospective multi-center randomized study comparing mobile cardiac outpatient telemetry versus standard loop event monitoring. *J Cardiovasc Electrophysiol* 2007;**18**:241–7.

13 Olson JA, Fouts AM, Padanilam BJ, *et al*. Utility of mobile cardiac outpatient telemetry for the diagnosis of palpitations, presyncope, syncope, and the assessment of therapy efficacy. *J Cardiovasc Electrophysiol* 2007;**18**:1–5.

14 Shen W, Decker W, Smars P. Syncope Evaluation in the Emergency Department Study (SEEDS): a multidisciplinary approach to syncope management. *Circulation* 2004;**110**:3636–45.

15 Quinn J, McDermott D, Stiell I, *et al*. Prospective validation of the San Francisco Syncope Rule to predict patients with serious outcomes. *Ann Emerg Med* 2006;**47**:448–54.

16 Sun BC, Mangione CM, Merchant G. External validation of the San Francisco Syncope Rule. *Ann Emerg Med* 2007;**49**:420–7.

17 Brignole M, Menozzi C, Bartoletti A. A new management of syncope: prospective systematic guideline-based evaluation of patients referred urgently to general hospitals. *Eur Heart J* 2006;**27**:76–82.

18 Brignole M, Ungar A, Bartoletti A. Standardized-care pathway versus usual management of syncope patients referred in emergency to general hospitals. *Europace* 2006;**8**:644–50.

19 Sauer A, Moss A, McNitt S, *et al*. Long QT syndrome in adults. *J Am Coll Cardiol* 2007;**49**:329–37.

20 Sacher F, Probst V, Iesaka Y, *et al*. Outcome after implantation of a cardioverter-defibrillator in patients with Brugada syndrome: a multicenter study. *Circulation* 2006;**114**:2317–24.

21 Andrea Sarkozy A, Boussy T, Kourgiannides G, *et al.* Long-term follow-up of primary prophylactic implantable cardioverter-defibrillator therapy in Brugada syndrome. *Eur Heart J* 2007;**28**:334–44.

22 Paul M, Schulze-Bahr E, Gerss J, *et al.* Impact of programmed ventricular stimulation in patients with Brugada syndrome: a meta-analysis of worldwide published data [abstract]. *Eur Heart J* 2006;**27**:470.

23 Alboni P, Brignole M, Degli Uberti E. Is vasovagal syncope a disease? *Europace* 2007;**9**:83–7.

24 Serletis A, Rose S, Sheldon AG, Sheldon RS. Vasovagal syncope in medical students and their first-degree relatives. *Eur Heart J* 2006;**27**:1965–70.

CHAPTER 28

Syncope and transient loss of consciousness: multidisciplinary management

A John Camm

Introduction

A multitude of mechanisms may cause transient loss of consciousness (TLOC); syncope is a specific form of TLOC that is related to a critical and reversible reduction of oxygenated blood flow to the brain. Metabolic problems, psychogenic causes such as hysteria, and primary neurological events such as an epileptic incident, are other causes of real or apparent TLOC that may closely simulate syncope. Cardiologists (arrhythmologists and hemodynamicists), clinical neurologists (especially autonomic neurologists), and psychiatrists may be needed to accurately diagnose and effectively manage patients presenting with transient loss of consciousness. A very wide range of often complex and expensive investigations must be available in order to facilitate diagnosis and an extensive pharmacopoeia, and a broad variety of therapies must be accessible to ensure successful treatment.

Syncope patients tend to present first to emergency room physicians, family practitioners, pediatricians, geriatricians, or general physicians who not surprisingly have few of the specialty skills and specialist equipment necessary for comprehensive evaluation of the syncopal patient [1]. For these generalists the initial management of the syncopal patient presents a bewildering choice of preliminary investigations and a large selection of possible referral pathways. Often the wrong choice will delay and compromise the effective diagnosis and management of the patient. When a syncopal patient is referred to a cardiac arrhythmologist, a train of investigations designed to expose cardiac arrhythmias that might be responsible for the syncope may be initiated irrespective of clinical clues as to the most likely cause of the event. Similarly, a neurologist will tend to concentrate on evaluating possible cerebral causes of TLOC, etc. Time and money are wasted; the patient is exposed to the risks

Syncope and Transient Loss of Consciousness, 1st edition. Edited by David G Benditt *et al*.
© 2007 Blackwell Publishing, ISBN: 978-1-4051-7625-5.

(a)

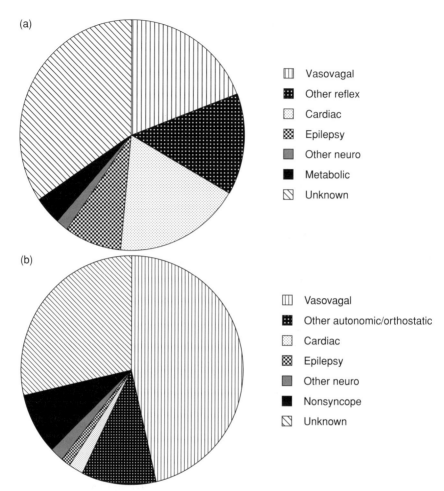

(b)

Figure 28.1 (a) Compilation of the causes of syncope from three series of patients (870 patients) compiled by Fitzpatrick and Cooper [2]. (b) Distribution of causes of syncope after assessment by neurologists of syncopal patients without an apparent ECG or clinical cardiac cause of syncope [3].

of possibly unnecessary investigations and potentially dangerous mistakes in the diagnosis. Despite this, whichever specialty takes responsibility for investigating, neurally-mediated syncope and "reflex" mechanisms proves to be the most common cause [2, 3] (Figure 28.1).

Misdiagnosis is common; for example, mechanical falls are misdiagnosed as syncope, syncope due to cardiac arrhythmia is misdiagnosed as epilepsy, and transient ischemic attacks are misdiagnosed as syncope. A particular dangerous problem has been the misdiagnosis of cardiac arrhythmias related to the long QT syndrome as being epileptic in nature. Many such patients were mistreated for years because antiepileptic drugs are of little value and in some instance might even aggravate cardiac arrhythmia related to long QT syndrome.

Situational syncope and other forms of neurocardiogenic syncope are often ignored or dismissed as unimportant by generalists. Patients with neurally-mediated reflex syncope who may also suffer from a range of associated autonomic disorders (irritable bowel syndrome, effort syndrome, etc.) may even be referred for psychiatric assessment when the cause of their syncope is easily discernible.

The solution to these problems lies in the provision of efficient diagnostic and management protocols and appropriate care pathways. The approach must be designed to access the skills and expertise of multiple disciplines—a team approach is the way forward.

Multidisciplinary clinic

There have been attempts to establish clinics that are staffed by members of several disciplines important to the accurate diagnosis of patients presenting with TLOC, particularly cardiology and neurology. Such clinics in the United Kingdom have been known as "blackout clinics," and rapid-access forms of these clinics have been established primarily to deal with the important evaluation of the initial presentation of epilepsy or "first fits." It often proves very difficult to align both cardiology and neurology services, and it should be appreciated that this is largely unnecessary since the majority of TLOC due to neurological causes can easily be distinguished from high-risk cardiology problems by simple clinical assessment. In most instances neurally-mediated syncope is obvious but the distinction between this and nonautonomic neurological causations of syncope and arrhythmia or occult cardiac disease may be difficult. It is therefore necessary for both neurologists and cardiologists to have access to autonomic investigations, especially tilt-table testing. An expert in autonomic neurology may significantly improve the quality of a multidisciplinary syncope service, and expert psychiatrists, metabolists, pulmonologists, etc., may also add value. However, it serves little or no purpose in trying to include all such specialists in joint clinics.

Shen *et al.* [4] reported a comparison between a novel syncope assessment unit and a standard medical care in 103 consecutive patients presenting to the emergency room with syncope of intermediate risk, but not loss of consciousness due to stroke or epilepsy. The syncope assessment involved collaboration between emergency room physicians, cardiologists, and electrophysiologists. The syncope unit offered clinical evaluation, 6-hour electrocardiogram (ECG), real-time monitoring, carotid sinus hypersensitivity testing, head-up tilt-testing echocardiography, and an electrophysiology consult. The diagnostic yield of the special syncope unit was 67% compared with 10% of patients who followed the conventional clinical pathway. Hospitalization was significantly reduced (from 98 to 43%). However, long-term survival and long-term freedom from syncope were not improved.

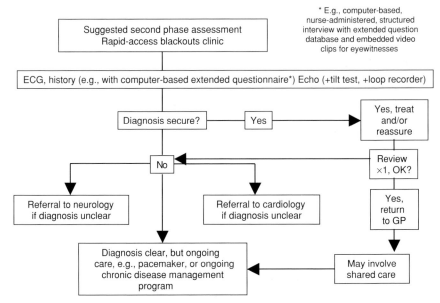

Figure 28.2 Point-of-care rapid access to blackouts clinic developed and approved by the Department of Health Expert Reference Group on Cardiac Arrhythmias and Sudden Cardiac Death (see [5]).

Nurse-led rapid-access syncope clinic

Triage systems with defined preliminary assessments, perhaps administered by nursing rather than physician personnel, may be a helpful approach to standardizing a rapid-access syncope service. Simple clinical criteria, mostly derived from the history of the patient and the TLOC event(s), may be used to classify patients as "likely" to have suffered cardiac, neurally-mediated, orthostatic, or nonsyncopal TLOC. Basic physical examination (cardiac and carotid auscultation, carotid sinus massage, and palpation of the pulse), inspection of the standard 12-lead ECG, and measurement of the blood pressure (lying and standing) will further refine the allocation of patients between these categories. Appropriate per protocol (care pathway) referral can then be rapidly achieved. However, a significant proportion of syncope will remain unexplained, and in such cases an initial evaluation for neurally-mediated syncope is advised, since this is by far the most likely cause and testing for this possibility that can easily be undertaken.

Health care payers, for example the UK Department of Health, have recognized the crucial importance of putting arrangements in place to effectively deal with syncope. Figure 28.2 is an example of the care pathway advocated by this government department; it stresses an evaluation that includes clinical assessment, tilt-table testing and loop recording, and appropriate referral to specific specialists, but acknowledges the need for specially designed protocols and, where necessary, shared care [5].

Care pathways

The standard clinical evaluation of syncope has been very substantially improved over the last decade. Much of this improvement is related to better understanding of the pathophysiology and mechanisms of syncope, particularly those attributable to autonomic disorders. Also, the more detailed evaluation of patients using autonomic function tests for the evaluation of neurally-mediated syncope and the more determined search for occult arrhythmias, for example, by early deployment of implantable loop recorders (ILRs), has led to improved diagnosis and management of this problem. All of this has resulted in a flurry of published recommendations for the management of syncope [6–9], including assessment of mortality risk [10]. However, guidelines alone do not improve management unless guideline implementation is ensured [11]. In order to facilitate this, management protocols or care pathways have been designed and introduced.

Ammirati and colleagues [12] reported the result of introducing a simple, two-step diagnostic algorithm for syncope. The first step was a baseline investigation comprising a detailed history and physical examination, 12-lead ECG, and glucose/hemoglobin dipstick measurements. The second step resulted from the most likely cause to emerge from the first step. The initial investigations in the second step were therefore focused on cardiac, neurally-mediated, or neuropsychiatric causes of syncope. Only if initial investigation failed were other causes targeted. Using this approach a "conclusive diagnosis" was reached before patient discharge in 87% compared with 65% prior to the introduction of this system.

Sarasin and colleagues [13] reported a similar two-stage method. Stage 1 comprised a standard evaluation, including history and physical examination, laboratory tests (hemoglobin, glucose, and creatine kinase), 12-lead ECG, orthostatic blood pressure measurement, and carotid sinus massage. A diagnosis was reached in 69% of patients at the end of this initial round. Stage 2 involved 24-hour electrocardiography, ambulatory loop monitoring, or electrophysiogical studies as determined by an abnormal 12-lead ECG, or a tilt-table test was performed to identify neurally-mediated syncope. After these tests an additional 8% of patients were diagnosed. Further Substantial investigation revealed only the cause of syncope in another 30 of the remaining 155 patients. Farwell and Sulke [14] further explored the "diagnostic hypothesis" and focused on investigation concept. They investigated 421 patients presenting with syncope and compared them with a retrospective series of 660 patients. Although the diagnostic yield increased only from 71 to 78%, the use of targeted resources fell significantly. However, the total cost of investigation per diagnosis rose significantly.

Conclusion

In previous times, a skilled general physician may have been sufficiently experienced and adequately available to manage patients with syncope. However, the diagnostic challenges and therapeutic strategies that are now available exceed the skills of any single medical practitioner. At present, it is agreed that it is necessary to adopt a multidisciplinary approach to syncope management in order to deal quickly, effectively, and cost-efficiently with this disorder that may result from so many causes. Otherwise, misdiagnoses and inappropriate therapies are inevitable.

Initially, it was felt that it might be necessary to arrange close collaborations between neurologists and cardiologists, but it is now appreciated that the majority of important neurology and cardiology conditions can be identified by a straightforward clinical evaluation together with an ECG and basic hematology/biochemistry measurements. Suitable protocols and care pathways can then direct prompt referral to the appropriate specialist who can arrange more targeted subsequent investigations that take advantage of the specialist techniques that are available only through that specialty. In this way the investigation of syncope achieves a high diagnostic yield in a cost-effective manner.

A more important multidisciplinary aspect to the management of syncope involves an alliance between emergency room physicians and those responsible for the investigation of cardiac and neurally-mediated syncope [15]. Neurological causes of TLOC are usually easy to spot, even though major neurological problems are a relatively unusual cause of true syncope. The majority of syncopal episodes are due to neurally-mediated mechanisms or inappropriate orthostatic blood pressure control. These mechanisms should be demonstrated and, wherever possible, diagnosed positively rather than presumptively.

In most centers, cardiologists or gerontologists with a special interest in cardiology or syncope are responsible for the investigation of syncope of autonomic origin. However, the diagnosis of cardiac arrhythmia or obstructive cardiac pathologies requires the specialist knowledge and expertise of the cardiologist. All in all, it has proven highly effective to develop an excellent relationship between emergency room staff, admitting physicians, or rapid-access blackout clinic triage nurses, and a cardiologist with a special interest in syncope. In addition, relevant care pathways and clinical protocols that point to appropriate referrals to other specialists should also be put in place to ensure the provision of a high-quality service for patients with syncope.

References

1 O'Connor J, Meurer LN. What is the diagnostic yield of a standardized sequential clinical evaluation of patients presenting to an emergency department with syncope? *J Fam Pract* 2001;**50**(12):1020.

2 Fitzpatrick AP, Cooper P. Diagnosis and management of patients with blackouts. *Heart* 2006;**92**;559–68.

3 Strano S, Colosimo C, Sparagna A, *et al.* Multidisciplinary approach for diagnosing syncope: a retrospective study on 521 outpatients. *J Neurol Neurosurg Psychiatry* 2005;**76**(11):1597–600.

4 Shen WK, Decker WW, Smars PA, *et al.* Syncope Evaluation in the Emergency Department Study (SEEDS): a multidisciplinary approach to syncope management. *Circulation* 2004;**110**(24):3636–45.

5 Developed and approved by the Department of Health Expert Reference Group on Cardiac Arrhythmias and Sudden Cardiac Death (NSF Chapter 8). Available at: http://www.dh.gov.uk/assetRoot/04/10/60/40/04106040.pdf.

6 Brignole M, Alboni P, Benditt DG, *et al.*; Task Force on Syncope, European Society of Cardiology. Guidelines on management (diagnosis and treatment) of syncope. *Eur Heart J* 2001;**22**(15):1256–306.

7 Brignole M, Alboni P, Benditt DG, *et al.*; Task Force on Syncope, European Society of Cardiology. Guidelines on management (diagnosis and treatment) of syncope. *Europace* 2004;**6**(6):467–537.

8 Strickberger SA, Benson DW, Biaggioni I, *et al.*; American Heart Association Councils on Clinical Cardiology, Cardiovascular Nursing, Cardiovascular Disease in the Young, and Stroke; Quality of Care and Outcomes Research Interdisciplinary Working Group; American College of Cardiology Foundation; Heart Rhythm Society; American Autonomic Society. AHA/ACCF Scientific Statement on the evaluation of syncope: from the American Heart Association Councils on Clinical Cardiology, Cardiovascular Nursing, Cardiovascular Disease in the Young, and Stroke, and the Quality of Care and Outcomes Research Interdisciplinary Working Group; and the American College of Cardiology Foundation in collaboration with the Heart Rhythm Society endorsed by the American Autonomic Society. *Circulation* 2006;**113**(2):316–27. Erratum in: *Circulation* 2006;**113**(14):e697.

9 Benditt DG; Ad Hoc Syncope Consortium. The ACCF/AHA Scientific Statement on Syncope: a document in need of thoughtful revision. *Europace* 2006;**8**(12):1017–21.

10 Colivicchi F, Ammirati F, Melina D, Guido V, Imperoli G, Santini M; OESIL (Osservatorio Epidemiologico sulla Sincope nel Lazio) Study Investigators. Development and prospective validation of a risk stratification system for patients with syncope in the emergency department: the OESIL risk score. *Eur Heart J* 2003;**24**(9):811–19.

11 Del Greco M, Cozzio S, Scillieri M, Caprari F, Scivales A, Disertori M. Diagnostic pathway of syncope and analysis of the impact of guidelines in a district general hospital: the ECSIT study (epidemiology and costs of syncope in Trento). *Ital Heart J* 2003;**4**(2):99–106.

12 Ammirati F, Colivicchi F, Santini M. Diagnosing syncope in clinical practice. Implementation of a simplified diagnostic algorithm in a multicentre prospective trial—the OESIL 2 study (Osservatorio Epidemiologico della Sincope nel Lazio). *Eur Heart J* 2000;**21**(11):935–40.

13 Sarasin FP, LouisSimonet M, Carballo D, *et al.* What is the diagnostic yield of a standardized sequential clinical evaluation of patients presenting to an emergency department with syncope? *J Fam Pract* 2001;**111**:177–84.

14 Farwell DJ, Sulke AN. Does the use of a syncope diagnostic protocol improve the investigation and management of syncope? *Heart* 2004;**90**(1):52–8.

15 Smars PA, Decker WW, Shen WK. Syncope evaluation in the emergency department. *Curr Opin Cardiol* 2007;**22**(1):44–8.

CHAPTER 29

Syncope practice guidelines initiative

David G Benditt

It is generally acknowledged that management of patients with real or apparent transient loss of consciousness (TLOC), of which syncope patients comprise an important subset, is not optimal. Multiple factors facing physicians and allied medical professionals contribute to this problem including:

• Inadequate appreciation of what TLOC is, its relationship to syncope, and the many potential causes of both.

• Insufficient understanding of the importance of a detailed medical history taking and the essential components of the history taking (including eyewitness accounts).

• Uncertainty regarding efficient and cost-effective diagnostic and treatment strategies.

• A tendency for medical specialties to work in isolation rather than as multidisciplinary units.

• Concern regarding exposure to medical–legal risk if comprehensive testing is not ordered, despite the increasingly recognized ineffectiveness of such a strategy.

European Society of Cardiology Syncope Guideline Initiative

In an attempt to provide an evidence-based direction for the TLOC/syncope evaluation, the European Society of Cardiology (ESC) commissioned development of syncope practice guidelines. This multidisciplinary, multinational effort resulted in publication of an initial guideline statement in 2001 [1] and a revised version in 2004 [2]. However, unfortunately at the time the ESC did not appreciate the virtue of attempting to broaden the guideline initiative to incorporate other professional organizations. Thus, despite the fact that noncardiology specialties such as neuroscience, internal medicine, and pediatrics were represented during the ESC guideline development, official endorsement of the ESC product was neither sought from nor provided by European societies of neurology, internal medicine, or pediatrics. Emergency medicine, geriatrics, and psychiatry (specialties that are relevant in a

Syncope and Transient Loss of Consciousness, 1st edition. Edited by David G Benditt *et al*.
© 2007 Blackwell Publishing, ISBN: 978-1-4051-7625-5.

broad-based TLOC/syncope guideline initiative) were not officially represented on the task force. Furthermore, the ESC declined to request that non-European professional societies participate, although the task force proposed that the Heart Rhythm Society (then called North America Society of Pacing and Electrophysiology) be invited to contribute on an official basis. As a consequence, by virtue of its being developed and published in Europe without the "official" input of a broad range of medical specialties, the ESC guidelines impact has been less than might have been the case. Indeed, the ESC guideline carries essentially no authority in North America other than as a comprehensive reference. In essence, the ESC guideline, while the most complete document of its kind, is inherently limited in its applicability to European cardiovascular specialists and the patients referred to them.

The need for greater physician education and a more well-organized approach to TLOC/syncope has been recognized as an important clinical issue in North America by several professional societies. The American College of Emergency Physicians and the American College of Physicians were the first to publish recommendations regarding care of such patients [3–5]. More recently, the American College of Cardiology (ACCF), the American Heart Association (AHA), the Heart Rhythm Society (HRS), and the American Autonomic Society have taken an interest in the problem. In this context, ACCF and AHA apparently determined that a consensus "scientific statement" was an appropriate and sufficient step to take, rather than a more extensive and expensive formal practice guideline initiative. Thus, the ACCF/AHA Syncope Statement [6] was launched. This statement unfortunately proved to be poorly crafted and controversial (see below). Nevertheless, despite its not being intended to be a formal set of practice guidelines and its being replete with deficiencies (many of which have been the subject of criticism [7, 8]), for many practitioners the ACCF/AHA Statement may be erroneously considered authoritative.

ACCF/AHA Syncope Statement deficiencies

Criticisms of the ACCF/AHA Syncope Statement have appeared on Heart.org, in *Journal of the American College of Cardiology* [7], and simultaneously in the journals *Europace* and *Clinical Autonomic Research* [8]. The source of these critiques is a multidisciplinary/multinational Ad Hoc Syncope Consortium, comprising in excess of 60 physicians (see Appendix) interested in management of TLOC/syncope patients. In large measure the Consortium was formed with the goals of publicizing the Statement's flaws and encouraging its careful revision; however, it also holds as a long-term goal, promoting development of comprehensive multidisciplinary practice guidelines.

With respect to ACCF/AHA Syncope Statement [6], the Consortium argued that the Statement had too many failings to be considered a credible reflection of the "state of the art." In brief, it did not provide readers with a clear understanding of the TLOC/ syncope problem in terms of proper definitions, evaluation priorities, or treatment strategy. Additionally, a large body

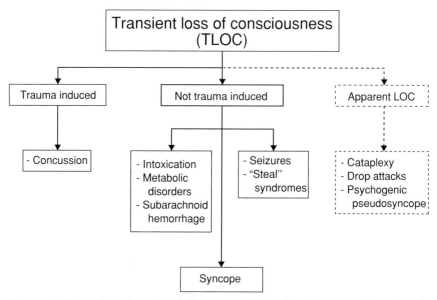

Figure 29.1 Schematic depicting the principal causes of TLOC. Note that syncope is a subset of TLOC.

of recent literature that should have been used to support any proposed recommendations was absent, thereby further diminishing the credibility of the document.

In terms of definitions, before a proper evaluation can begin, clinicians need to be provided a clear understanding of the fundamental issue, "what is syncope?" The ACCF/AHA Statement does not establish the distinction between "syncope" and the broader problem of TLOC (Figure 29.1). Specifically, TLOC, apart from syncope, includes such diverse conditions as concussion due to trauma, epileptic seizures due to a primary electrical problem in the brain, and "apparent TLOC," such as that may occur with conversion disorders. Absence of a clear understanding of the problems at hand inevitably leads to excessive and generally futile overuse of diagnostic tests.

With regard to clinical priorities, the ACCF/AHA Statement focused its concerns on mortality issues associated with syncope rather than the broader problem of optimal patient care. The authors indicated that the primary "purpose of the (syncope) evaluation" is "to determine whether the patient is at increased risk for death." As a consequence of this bias, the statement targeted the relatively small, albeit important, subset of high-risk patients (perhaps 20% of those with syncope who may require treatment with cardiovascular interventions, including medications, implantable cardioverter-defibrillators (ICDs), or pacemakers) and underemphasized the far more prevalent causes of syncope, such as those of neurally-mediated reflex or orthostatic origin. The reality is that for the vast majority of patients with presumed syncope, the underlying causes confer not so much a life-threatening risk as a diminished quality of life, or an increased potential for physical injury and economic risk. These latter issues are crucial to well-being. Consequently, the rationale for the syncope evaluation must be a more *fundamental* one, namely, to establish the cause symptoms with sufficient confidence to assess prognosis and recommend an effective treatment strategy.

Among the more surprising failings of the ACCF/AHA Statement was absence of a strong supportive evidence base for its positions. Many pertinent contributions to the TLOC/syncope evaluation literature were overlooked, including citation of either of the two ESC syncope practice guideline publications [1, 2]. Further, among other important missing works was either of the two major North American pacing trials targeting syncope patients [9, 10], an important beta-blocker trial [11, 12], or the only extant trial examining the utility of an organized syncope management unit in a North American hospital [13]. The statement failed to cite most of the many published European randomized and/or controlled clinical trials that assessed various aspects of syncope evaluation and treatment. With the exception of SAFE-PACE [14], published clinical trials such as EGSYS [15], OESIL [16] and OESIL2 [17], ISSUE-1 [18–20], VASIS [21, 22], SYDIT [23], and SYNPACE [24] were not cited.

Despite its inadequacies, publication of the ACCF/AHA Statement provides evidence of concern in North America regarding the need for improving TLOC/syncope management.

Potential utility of a multidisciplinary practice guideline

In order for a practice guideline to direct medical care appropriately in a field as broad as TLOC/syncope, it must receive input and official acceptance from a wide range of caregivers (e.g., cardiologists, neurologists, internal medicines, pediatrics, and geriatrics). Development of such a multidisciplinary, multinational TLOC/syncope practice guideline would be unique, and the effort and expense would not be trivial. However, preliminary experience with the ESC product suggests that substantial benefit (in both clinical and economic terms) can be expected. In this regard, two published studies provide supportive evidence; each compared the impact of a "guided" care approach to the TLOC/syncope evaluation with a preceding period of "usual" care.

OESIL [16] evaluated "usual" care outcomes associated with emergency room visits and hospitalizations for syncope in 15 Rome hospitals during a 2-month period. Among 781 patients included in the study, 450 were hospitalized (58%) for an average of 7 days. A cardiovascular cause was reported in 34% and noncardiovascular causes in 12%. Most importantly, the cause remained unknown in 54% of cases. Subsequently, OESIL-2 [17] reevaluated outcomes after introducing a relatively simple algorithm to direct care. During the reassessment, the cause was determined to be cardiovascular in 21%, neural-reflex in 35%, and noncardiovascular in 14%. Of note, unknown cases dropped to 14%.

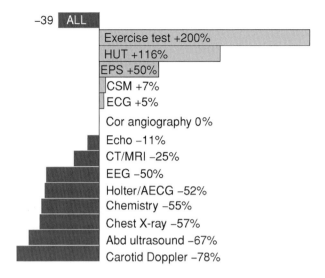

Figure 29.2 Impact of "standardized care" on diagnostic testing selection. The abcissa indicates percent increase or decrease of the specific test in "standardized care" versus "usual care" groups. (Modified after Brignole *et al.* [26].)

An even more comprehensive evaluation of standardized methodology was reported in the Evaluation of Guidelines in Syncope Study 2 (EGSYS-2) [25, 26]. In this prospective, controlled, multicenter study, the ESC Syncope Guidelines formed the basis for standardized care. Findings in patients referred to 19 Italian general hospitals and managed according to the standardized care pathway were compared with findings obtained in patients managed according to usual practice. The two groups comprised 929 patients in usual care and 745 patients in standardized care. At the end of the evaluation, the standardized care group had a 17% lower hospitalization rate, 11% shorter in-hospital stay, 26% fewer tests performed per patient (median 2.5 vs 3.4), and fewer patients being labeled as unexplained syncope (5% vs 20% in the usual care group). Further, the total number of diagnostic tests was reduced by 39%, as were the number of low-yield tests (as identified by the ESC Syncope Guidelines, e.g., brain scans and EEGs) (Figure 29.2). The mean cost per patient was 19% lower (€1127 vs €1394), and the mean cost per diagnosis was 29% lower (€1240 vs €1753), in the standardized care group. Thus, a standardized care pathway based on a broadly accepted guideline offers the potential for substantial clinical and economic benefit.

Despite the apparent value of preparing well-considered guidelines, putting them into clinical practice will be a challenge, but a necessary one. By way of illustration, a recent study examined one of the most important issues facing physicians responsible for initial care of patients thought to have suffered syncope. Specifically, "does this individual need in-hospital evaluation?" The

Table 29.1 When to hospitalize a patient with syncope for diagnostic evaluation.*

Strongly recommended for diagnosis
   Suspected or known significant heart disease
   ECG abnormalities suggestive of arrhythmic syncope
   Syncope occurring during exercise
   Syncope causing severe injury
   Strong family history of sudden death

Occasionally may need to be admitted
   Patients with or without heart disease but with:
     • sudden onset of palpitations shortly before syncope
     • syncope in supine position
     • worrisome family history
     • significant physical injury
   Patients with minimal or mild heart disease when there is high suspicion for cardiac syncope
   Suspected pacemaker or ICD problem

*Based on ESC Syncope Task Force Guidelines [1, 2].

outcome of this decision has many implications, including lifestyle and economic concerns for the patient, as well as health care management issues (e.g., bed availability, hospital costs, and laboratory utilization). The ESC Syncope Task Force expended considerable effort on this topic [1, 2] (Table 29.1).

Recently, Bartoletti *et al.* [27] addressed the question whether emergency department physicians appropriately elected hospitalization or outpatient evaluation in a group of patients presenting with TLOC/syncope. The physicians were trained with respect to the ESC guidelines, and particularly in regard to hospital admission recommendations. During the approximate 2-year enrollment period, 1124 patients were deemed to have had a true syncope, and 440 of these (39%) had at least one marker supporting admission for evaluation; 393 of these 440 patients (89%) were admitted. On the other side of the coin, 684 patients met no evident admission criterion; 511 of 684 patients (75%) were appropriately discharged from the emergency department (presumably for out-of-hospital evaluation), but 25% were nonetheless admitted. These results are encouraging. The 25% admission rate in low-risk patients is probably less than is generally the case in practice; nonetheless, it indicates that, despite being "backed up" by a guideline statement, emergency department physicians preferred to "err" on the side of admission and observation. Clearly, apart from formulating guidelines, agencies must take a proactive stance to assure their effective application in practice [28].

Conclusion

The management of patients who present after an apparent TLOC/syncope episode has long been a clinical challenge, and clinical guidelines are clearly needed. In this regard, the ESC published the first set of guidelines on the management (diagnosis and treatment) of syncope in 2001, with the most recent update being issued in 2004 [1]. Nevertheless, despite the fact that the ESC recommendations are the most comprehensive statements addressing the optimal approach to the TLOC/syncope patient currently available, and several studies support their effectiveness, their applicability remains limited primarily to cardiovascular specialists in Europe. A guideline having broader acceptance is needed. To this end, the recent interest and controversy generated by the ACCF/AHA Statement may prove helpful. Potentially, key professional organizations will recognize both the need for guidelines that are applicable across the many specialties that care for TLOC/syncope patients and the benefits of a cooperative multidisciplinary approach to guideline development.

References

1 Brignole M, Alboni P, Benditt DG, *et al*. Guidelines on management (diagnosis and treatment) of syncope. *Eur Heart J* 2001;**22**:1256–306.

2 Brignole M, Alboni P, Benditt DG, *et al*. Guidelines on management (diagnosis and treatment) of syncope—update 2004. *Europace* 2004;**6**:467–537.

3 American College of Emergency Physicians. Clinical policy: critical issues in the evaluation and management of patients presenting with syncope. *Ann Emerg Med* 2001;**37**:771–6.

4 Linzer M, Yang E, Estes M, *et al*. Clinical guideline: diagnosing syncope. Part 1: Value of history, clinical examination, and electrocardiography. *Ann Intern Med* 1997;**126**:989–96.

5 Linzer M, Yang E, Estes M, *et al*. Clinical guideline: diagnosing syncope. Part 2: Unexplained syncope. *Ann Intern Med* 1997;**127**:76–86.

6 Strickberger SA, Benson DW, Jr, Biaggioni I, *et al*. AHA/ACCF scientific statement on the evaluation of syncope. *J Am Coll Cardiol* 2006;**47**:473–84; *Circulation* 2006;**113**:316–27.

7 Benditt DG, Olshansky B, Wieling W; on behalf of the Ad Hoc Syncope Consortium. The ACCF/AHA Scientific Statement on Syncope needs rethinking [letter]. *J Am Coll Cardiol* 2006;**48**(12):2598–9.

8 Benditt DG; on behalf of the Ad Hoc Syncope Consortium. The ACCF/AHA Scientific Statement on Syncope: a document in need of thoughtful revision. *Europace* 2006;**8**:1017–21; *Clin Auton Res* 2006;**16**:363–8.

9 Connolly SJ, Sheldon R, Roberts RS, Gent M; Vasovagal Pacemaker Study Investigators. The North American Vasovagal Pacemaker Study (VPS): a randomized trial of permanent cardiac pacing for the prevention of vasovagal syncope. *J Am Coll Cardiol* 1999;**33**:16–20.

10 Connolly S, Sheldon R, Thorpe KE, *et al*. Pacemaker therapy for prevention of syncope in patients with recurrent vasovagal syncope. *JAMA* 2003;**289**:2224–9.

11 Sheldon R, Rose S, Connolly S. Prevention of Syncope Trial (POST): a randomized clinical trial of beta blockers in the prevention of vasovagal syncope. Rationale and study design. *Europace* 2003;**5**:71–5.

12 Sheldon RS, Connelly S, Rose S, *et al*. The Prevention of Syncope Trial (POST): a randomized, placebo-controlled study of metoprolol in the prevention of vasovagal syncope. *Circulation* 2006;113:1164–70.

13 Shen WK, Decker WW, Smars PA, *et al*. Syncope Evaluation in the Emergency Department Study (SEEDS): a multidisciplinary approach to syncope management. *Circulation* 2004;**110**(24):3636–45.

14 Kenny RA, Richardson DA, Steen N, *et al.* Carotid sinus syndrome: a modifiable risk factor for non-accidental falls in older adults (SAFE PACE). *J Am Coll Cardiol* 2001;**38**(5): 1491–6.

15 Brignole M, Disertori M, Menozzi C, *et al.*; Evaluation of Guidelines in Syncope Study Group. Management of syncope referred urgently to general hospitals with and without syncope units. *Europace* 2003;**5**:293–8.

16 Ammirati F, Colivicchi F, Minardi G, *et al.* Hospital management of syncope: the OESIL study. *G Ital Cardiol* 1999;**29**:533–9.

17 Ammirati F, Colivicchi F, Santini M, *et al.* Diagnosing syncope in clinical practice: implementation of a simplified diagnostic algorithm in a multicentre prospective trial – the OESIL 2 study (Observatorio Epidemiologico della Sincope nel Lazio). *Eur Heart J* 2000;**21**:935–40.

18 Moya A, Brignole M, Menozzi C, *et al.*; ISSUE Investigators. Mechanism of syncope in patients with isolated syncope and in patients with tilt-positive syncope. *Circulation* 2001;**104**:1261–7.

19 Brignole M, Menozzi C, Moya A, *et al.* Mechanism of syncope in patients with bundle branch block and negative electrophysiologic test. *Circulation* 2001;104:2045–50.

20 Menozzi C, Brignole M, Garcia-Civera R, *et al.* Mechanism of syncope in patients with heart disease and negative electrophysiologic test. *Circulation* 2002;**105**:2741–5.

21 Raviele A, Brignole M, Sutton R, *et al.* Effect of etilefrine in preventing syncopal recurrence in patients with vasovagal syncope: a double-blind, randomized, placebo-controlled trial. The Vasovagal Syncope International Study. *Circulation* 1999;**99**(11):1452–57.

22 Sutton R, Brignole M, Menozzi C, *et al.*; VASIS Investigators. Dual-chamber pacing is efficacious in treatment of neurally-mediated tilt-positive cardioinhibitory syncope. Pacemaker versus no therapy: a multicentre randomized study. *Circulation* 2000;**102**:294–9.

23 Ammirati F, Colivicchi F, Santini M, *et al.* Permanent cardiac pacing versus medical treatment for the prevention of recurrent vasovagal syncope: a multicenter, randomized, controlled trial. *Circulation* 2001;**104**:52–6.

24 Raviele A, Giada F, Menozzi C, *et al.*; Vasovagal Syncope and Pacing Trial Investigators. A randomized, double-blind, placebo-controlled study of permanent cardiac pacing for the treatment of recurrent tilt-induced vasovagal syncope. The Vasovagal Syncope and Pacing Trial (SYNPACE). *Eur Heart J* 2004;**25**:1741–8.

25 Brignole M, Menozi C, Bartoletti A, *et al.* A new management of syncope: prospective systematic guideline-based evaluation of patients referred urgently to general hospitals. *Eur Heart J* 2006;**27**:76–82.

26 Brignole M, Ungar A, Bartoletti A, *et al.* Standardized-care pathway vs usual management of syncope patients presenting as emergencies at general hospitals. *Europace* 2006;**8**:644–50.

27 Bartoletti A, Fabiani P, Adriani P, *et al.* Hospital admission of patients referred to the emergency department for syncope: a single-hospital prospective study based on the application of the European Society of Cardiology guidelines on syncope. *Eur Heart J* 2006;**27**:83–8.

28 Benditt DG. Syncope management guidelines at work: first steps towards assessing clinical utility. *Eur Heart J* 2006;**27**:7–9.

Appendix: syncope consortium members

Haruhiko Abe, MD, FACC
University of Occupational and Environmental Health, Kitakyushu, Japan

Paolo Alboni, MD
Ospedale Civile, Cento, Italy

Dietrich Andresen, MD, FESC
Vivantes-Klinikum Am Urban/Im Friedrichshain, Berlin, Germany

Felicia B Axelrod, MD
New York University School of Medicine, New York, USA

David G Benditt, MD, FACC, FRCP(C), FHRS (Correspondence)
University of Minnesota Medical School, Minnesota

Eduardo Bennaroch, MD
Mayo Clinic, Rochester, Minnesota, USA

Lennart Bergfeldt, MD, PhD, FESC
Sahlgrenska University Hospital, Gothenburg, Sweden

Jean Jacques Blanc, MD, FESC
Universite de Brest, Brest, France

Michele Brignole, MD, FESC
Ospedali del Tigullio, Lavagna, Italy

A John Camm, MD, FRCP, FACC, FESC
St George's Medical School of London, London, UK

Thomas Chelimsky, MD
University Hospitals of Cleveland, Cleveland, Ohio, USA

Pietro Cortelli, MD
Alma Mater Studiorum-Universita'di Bologna, Bologna, Italy

J Gert van Dijk, MD, PhD
Leiden University Medical Centre, Leiden, The Netherlands

Nynke van Dijk, MD
University of Amsterdam, Amsterdam, The Netherlands

Hugo Ector, MD, FESC
University Hospital, Leuven. Belgium

Cengiz Ermis, MD
Akendiz University, Antalya, Turkey

Murray Esler, MD
Baker Heart Research Institute, Melbourne, Australia

Adam Fitzpatrick, MD, FESC
Manchester Heart Centre, Manchester, UK

Fetnat Fouad-Tarazi, MD, FACC
Cleveland Clinic Foundation, Cleveland, Ohio, USA

Roy Freeman, MD
Beth Israel Deaconess Medical Center, Boston, Massachusetts, USA

Nora Goldschlager, MD, FACC, FHRS
University of California-San Francisco, USA

MaryAnn Goldstein, MD
Pediatric Emergency Medicine, Minneapolis, Minnesota, USA

Blair Grubb, MD FACC
Medical College of Ohio, Toledo, Ohio, USA

Prof. Roger Hainsworth
Leeds, United Kingdom

Bengt Herweg, MD
University of South Florida, Tampa, Florida, USA

Max J Hilz, MD, PhD
University Erlangen-Nuremberg, Erlangen, Germany

Giris Jacob, MD, DSc
Rambam Medical Center and Technion IIT, Hiafa, Israel

David Jardine, MD, FRACP
Christchurch School of Medicine, University of Otago, Christchurch, New Zealand

Jens Jordan, MD
Charité Campus Buch, Berlin, Germany

Michael J Joyner, MD
Mayo Clinic, Rochester, Minnesota, USA

Wishwa Kapoor, MD, MPH
University of Pittsburgh, Pittsburgh, Pennsylvania, USA

Horacio Kaufmann, MD
Mount Sinai School of Medicine, New York, USA

Rose-Anne Kenny, MD, FESC
Trinity College, Dublin 2, Ireland

Andrew Krahn, MD, FRCPC, FACC, FACP
University of Western Ontario, London, Ontario, Canada

Chu-Pak Lau, MBBS, MD, MRCP, FRCP, FACC, FRCP, FRACP, FESC
Hong Kong University and Queen Mary Hospital, Hong Kong, China

Benjamin D Levine, MD, FACC, FACSM
University of Texas Southwestern Medical Center at Dallas, Texas, USA

Johannes J van Lieshout, MD, PhD
University of Amsterdam, Amsterdam, The Netherlands

Mark Linzer, MD
University of Wisconsin, Madison, Wisconsin, USA

Lewis Lipsitz, MD
Harvard Medical School, Beth Israel Deaconess Medical Center, Boston, Massachusetts, USA

Philip Low, MD
Mayo Clinic, Rochester, Minnesota, USA

Keith G Lurie, MD, FACC
University of Minnesota Medical School and Central Minnesota Heart Center
 Minneapolis and St Cloud, Minnesota, USA

Marek Malik, Phd
St George's Hospital, London, UK

Christopher J Mathias, DPhil DSc, FRCP, FMedSci
University College London, London, UK

Angel Moya, MD, FESC
Hospital General Vall d'Hebron, Barcelona, Spain

Brian Olshansky, MD, FACC
University of Iowa Medical School, Iowa City, Iowa, USA

Oscar Oseroff, MD, FACC
Buenos Aires, Argentina

Satish R Raj, MD
Vanderbilt University, Nashville, Tennessee, USA

Antonio Raviele, MD, FESC
Ospedale Umberto I, Mestre-Venice, Italy

Sanjeev Saksena, MD, FACC, FESC
Robert Wood Johnson Medical School, Millburn, New Jersey, USA

Francois P Sarasin, MD, MSc
University of Geneva Medical School, Geneva, Switzerland

Philip J Saul, MD, FACC
Medical University of South Carolina, Charleston, South Carolina, USA

Ronald Schondorf, PhD, MD, FRCP(C)
McGill University, Montreal, Quebec, Canada

Jean-Michel Senard, MD
University of Toulouse, Toulouse, France

Robert Sheldon, MD, PhD, FRCP(C)
University of Calgary, Calgary, Alberta, Canada

Win-Kuang Shen, MD, FACC
Mayo Clinic, Rochester, Minnesota, USA

Jasbir Sra, MD, FACC
University of Wisconsin, Milwaukee, Wisconsin, USA

John Stephenson, BA, BM BCh, MA, DM (Oxford)
Royal Hospital for Sick Children, Glasgow, UK

Julian M Stewart, MD, PhD
New York Medical College, Hawthorne, New York, USA

Richard Sutton, DScMed, FRCP, FESC, FACC
Imperial College of London, London, UK

Hidetaka Tanaka, MD, PhD
Osaka Medical College Hospital, Osaka, Japan

George Theodorakis, MD, FESC
Onassis Cardiac Surgery Center, Athens, Greece

Roland D Thijs, MD, Phd
Leiden University Medical Center, Leiden, The Netherlands

Andrea Ungar, MD, PhD
University of Florence, Florence, Italy

Wouter Wieling, MD, PhD
University of Amsterdam, Amsterdam, The Netherlands

AAM Wilde, MD, PhD
Academic Medical Center Amsterdam, Amsterdam, The Netherlands

Index